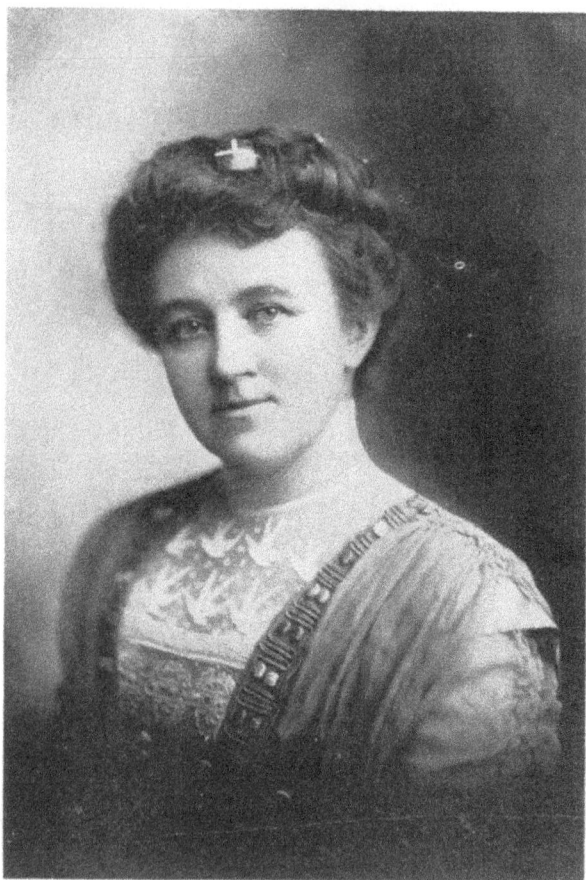

Susanna Cocroft.

What to Eat and When

By

Susanna Cocroft

Author of
"Let's Be Healthy," "The Woman Worth While"
"Growth in Silence," etc.

Fourth Edition

With Additions and Revisions to Date

Illustrated

G. P. Putnam's Sons
New York and London
The Knickerbocker Press
1916

The Knickerbocker Press, New York

PREFACE

THE subject of dietetics has only of late years begun to come into its own. For centuries it was thought that the body was a thing to be neglected and despised; that it was a clog to the soul. The teachings of dogma and the life of the hermit and the ascetic glorified the mortification of the body and the elevation of the soul.

The study of the functions of life and the manner in which those functions are upheld and vivified—the development of the sciences of Biology and Physiology—have placed the relations of the body and its inhabitant the soul on a more consistent and rational basis. It is coming to be recognized that the mind cannot function to its highest efficiency in a body below par; that in order to work harmoniously and to accomplish the most for humanity, the sound mind must dwell in a sound body, with all of its functions active, its organs in vigorous condition, kept so by a thorough assimilation and a forceful circulation. These are to be secured by means of daily exercise, abundance of fresh air, and healthful, happy, constructive thoughts.

It has been well said that the distinguishing feature between man and other animals is the fact that he is a cooking animal. Until he discovered fire man's subsistence was little more than that of the brute.

iii

Out of his discovery of the varied uses of this element came modern civilization. Much of this advance was made possible through the added strength of mind that was given man by a more varied diet. His limited raw diet gave little scope to his inventive faculties. From the discovery of the possibilities in cooked food his mind was stimulated to research in other directions. With the lessened need for vigorous mastication, however, the degeneration of man's teeth began and we are slowly learning now that exercise for the teeth and gums is as necessary for their health as it is for the rest of the body.

Dietetics is, in itself, both an Art and a Science. Food can be prepared so tastefully and its appearance made so pleasing as to become a fit subject for a painter. But the selection of food that shall give the body all the elements it needs in its work of growth and repair, with the greatest economy of effort, of purse, of time, and of energy, needs the trained judgment, the knowledge of comparative values and of chemical combinations possessed by a scientist. This is especially true from the fact that so many bodily ills result from a faulty digestion, due either to the food itself or to the condition of the organs which must handle the food.

The subject is so vast and its ramifications so many that all the resources of chemistry own themselves baffled at some of its intricacies. However, an intelligent working knowledge of the processes undergone by food in its progress through the body, and its transformation into vital force, can be attained by anyone.

This book is the outcome of years of experience in **correcting** bodily ills caused by wrong hygienic

Preface

habits. It has been written out of a sincere desire to awaken the every-day individual to the important relation that food bears to his well-being.

Much has been written on this subject by medical men for the medical profession, in language too technical for the layman. It is believed that in this book the layman will find a fund of information hitherto not available to him, in language stripped of technicalities, plain and easily understood. I have tried to make it logical and interesting.

When the American people become convinced that a thing is needed they generally "go after" it, and sooner or later the desired thing is attained. When they arouse themselves to see that the food they eat is pure, well prepared, and taken into digestive systems vigorous by means of proper exercise and fresh air, a new and far more virile race will be the outcome.

Acknowledgment is here made of the valuable assistance of Winfield S. Hall, Ph.D., M.D., Professor of Physiology in the Northwestern Medical School, Lecturer, and Author of *Nutrition and Dietetics;* of Alida Frances Pattee, late Instructor in Dietetics, Bellevue Training School for Nurses, Bellevue Hospital, New York City, Author of *Practical Dietetics.*

The tables of Food Values and the classification of foods are kindly furnished by Dr. Hall and used by the courtesy of his publishers, while a few of the recipes are generously furnished by Miss Pattee. Recognition is also made of the good work of Miss Helen Hammel, former dietitian in Wesley Hospital, Chicago, in the preparation of some of the recipes.

THE AUTHOR.

INTRODUCTION

THE problem of proper nutrition for the body is as vital as any study affecting the morals, health, and consequent power of a nation, since on the quality and quantity of food they assimilate, depend the sustenance, health, and strength of its citizens.

The food eaten by a nation largely determines the character of that nation.

No subject is so vital to the individual, to the family, the community, the nation, as health. No education is so vital as a knowledge of foods, sanitation, hygiene.

Health is the basis of happiness and the attainment of happiness is man's chief pursuit. The very foundation of national life is the education of its citizens in its preservation. The nation seeks prosperity and happiness—yet true prosperity is based on these fundamentals.

Money can be expended for no object which will yield the nation, or the individual, greater returns than in the acquisition of a knowledge of how to keep well. Health specialists, in the future, will direct their work more to the prevention than to the cure of diseases.

The strongest powers are those which most fully guard the health of their citizens. The endurance of an army lies in the strength of the individual soldier.

The basic work for "preparedness" is in building the bulwarks of physical strength and endurance.

The study of life is of most vital interest. The enjoyment and maintenance of life is inbred. It is intuitive. The infant's first instinct is the preservation of life; almost immediately he seeks for nourishment.

His body is an ever awakening wonder to him. He begins his education by testing his lungs, by studying his hands, his legs, and his flesh.

The human race spends more time in providing nourishment for the body than in any other line of activity. Yet we are wasteful; we have not studied to make the food yield its greatest nourishment and the body its greatest efficiency.

Unless the system is thoroughly nourished we miss much of the physical satisfaction of life; we miss the joys of mental development, the inspiration of soul, the sense of growth, of freedom, of expansion, and the self-satisfaction of accomplishing. The satisfaction resulting from greatest usefulness and the enjoyment of the results of usefulness, the greatest blessings and the largest measure of life come only to those whose nutriment is proper in quantity and quality, taken properly as to time, and is thoroughly assimilated, because both body and brain are thereby enabled to develop most fully.

The enjoyment of vibrant life, of bodily efficiency, is far beyond the fancied joys of the intemperate or the ascetic.

That one may thoroughly enjoy life in the freedom which comes from perfect activity of bodily functions, it is necessary that proper *habits* be formed, then the energy of thought is not constantly engaged in deciding what is best. Habit calls for no conscious expenditure of energy.

Nutrition is a broad subject. It means not only
that the foods be supplied which contain elements
required to rebuild body substance and to create heat
and energy, but it embraces, also, the ability of the
body to appropriate the foods to its needs.

The study of nutrition in its full sense, therefore,
must embrace not only foods, but anatomy and physiology (particularly of the digestive system). A
knowledge of chemistry is also necessary that we may
know the changes foods undergo in being converted
into tissue, heat, and energy.[1]   This science is known
as Dietetics.

Scientific research along the lines of electricity,
psychology, metaphysics, medicine, and art has been
tenaciously pursued for centuries; yet scientific study
of the natural means of keeping the body in health,
that the individual may be in physical, mental, and
moral condition to enjoy and to profit by researches
made in other lines, has been neglected.

The entire framework of the body—bone, muscle,
blood, brain, and nerve—as well as the heat and the
mental and physical energy necessary for every motion is supplied from food and drink, and from the
oxygen breathed into the lungs.

We are learning that derangements of the body are
largely caused by injudicious eating, yet, vital as it is,
the subject of foods, except in recent years, has not had
a place in the courses of study in our public schools.

[1] It is impossible in this book to go into the anatomy and
physiology of digestion exhaustively. The reader is respectfully
referred to Miss Cocroft's book on *Let's Be Healthy*. This traces
the food through the digestive canal, indicating the juices which
act on it, putting it into the state in which it can be absorbed by
the body and appropriated to its various uses.

We have given much attention to the "pound of cure," but insufficient attention to the "ounce of prevention." Man does not enjoy life to its full, nor do his physical or mental efforts yield him his best returns unless his system is thoroughly nourished.

Formerly, the physician gave general directions, or none at all, as to the diet. His directions, when given, were often indefinite because the subject was not definitely understood, due to the fact that the course of instruction in medical colleges contained practically nothing on the subject of foods. This study is not in the curriculum of all of our medical colleges to-day.

Our public-school curriculum contains no more important study than that of health and of the simple, hygienic laws which enable us to retain it. The science of foods in their relation to health, sanitation, and general hygiene should be among the foremost requirements of our public-school courses of study. Mothers' clubs will find no more interesting or profitable study than Dietetics.

It is coming to be widely recognized that a far larger number of diseases arise from the food habit than from the liquor habit. Many who look with contempt or pity on the victims of alcohol, are themselves diseased of body through the unintelligent use of food.

Habitual overeating not only produces diseases of the digestive organs, from overwork and excessive secretory activity, but also of the excretory and glandular system, as the kidneys and the liver, and may give rise to functional disturbances of the heart.

Food, if taken in greater quantity than the digestive juices can handle, either passes out of the system without being absorbed or it ferments or decomposes, giving rise to constipation, diarrhea, or other intestinal disturbances.

If the stomach and intestines are active and can handle the excess of food, its absorption beyond what the system requires overloads the blood and causes obesity or diseases of the skin and kidneys. It thus brings about abnormal deposits as in gout, or the calculi found in the kidney or the gall-bladder. Biliousness and congestion of the liver may follow, with constant headache, coated tongue, foul breath, and languor of body and of mind.

Many habitually eat too much and take too little fluid, though, due to a greater spread of knowledge, overeating is becoming less common.

On the other hand, an insufficient or illy balanced diet will bring in its train disorders of the system scarcely less harmful. A large number, particularly of young girls, take insufficient food, eat irregularly, and are undernourished.

When one does not eat sufficient food or the proper kind and variety, the tissues of the digestive organs are undernourished and do their work imperfectly.

The undernourished are usually those who work at high tension, those who worry, or those who do not get bodily exercise proportionate to the mental.

Mental workers are liable to become preoccupied and forget to take food. Growing girls who are over-interested in studies, anxious concerning examinations, etc., neglect their meals. Parents are often to blame in these cases by unduly encouraging the intellectual effort.

Members of some religious sects practice under-eating as a form of asceticism; many others from poverty are unable to procure a sufficient amount of food.

Too many, if not the majority of those concerned with the purchase and preparation of food, understand but little of food values and the importance of their proper combination. No matter how simple the menu, it should embrace the elements the system needs for its complete sustenance.

The problem of nutrition must be solved largely through chemistry. The health and efficiency of the individual and of the nation depend on careful study of the foods placed on the market, their chemical components, and their possible adulteration.

Happily the United States Government, realizing that its power as a nation depends on the strength and health of its citizens, has established experimental and analytical food departments. As a result of the findings of the government chemists, there was enacted in 1906, the Food and Drugs Act, which has raised the standard of food purity, by prescribing the conditions under which foods may be manufactured and sold. The law compels the maker of artificially colored or preserved food products to correctly label his goods. The national law instigated the passage of various state laws, which have further helped to insure a supply of pure food products; yet we need other laws which shall have greater efficiency and wider scope.

The strength of Germany as a nation is due very largely to the government supervision of foods manufactured and imported.

There is no more important branch of the United States Government than that which protects the health of its citizens.

The custom among some nations of retaining a physician to *maintain* the health of the family rather than to *regain* it, to *avoid* disease rather than to *cure* it, has its distinct advantages.

We should not be satisfied with anything less than perfect health and we are beginning to realize that this perfect health is a possibility for almost every individual.

In the maintenance of health, as well as in the cure of disease, diet is often more important than drugs.

To-day, scientific knowledge of hygiene and of food values is within the reach of all, and every mother and teacher may learn how to guard the health of those in her charge.

It is necessary to know the comparative values of foods as nutrient agents, in order to maintain our bodies in health and strength, and with economy of digestive effort, as well as efficiency.

There is no study, therefore, more important than that of bodily nutrition, which comprises not only the right proportion of food and drink, but also the manner in which they must be prepared in order to yield the best returns under varying conditions—age, employment, health, and sickness.

The body is certainly a marvelous machine! It is self-building, self-repairing, and, to a degree, self-regulating.

It appropriates to its use foodstuffs for growth and for repair.

It eliminates its waste.

It supplies the energy for rebuilding, and eliminating this waste.

It directs its own emotions.

It supplies the energy for these emotions.

It discriminates in the selection of food and casts out refuse and foodstuffs not needed.

It forms brain cells and creates mental force with which to control the organism.

It keeps in repair the nerves, which are the telegraph wires connecting the brain with all parts of the body.

It converts the potential energy in the food into heat with which to keep itself warm.

Withal it is not left entirely free to do its work automatically. It has within it a higher intelligence, a spiritual force, which may definitely hamper its workings by getting a wrong control of the telegraph wires, thus interfering with the digestion, the heart action, the lungs, and all metabolic changes. The right exercise of this higher intelligence, in turn, depends on the condition of the body, because when the mechanism of the body is out of repair it hampers mental and spiritual control.

About one-third of the food eaten goes to maintain the life of the body in its incessant work of repairing and rebuilding, the remaining two-thirds being held in reserve for other activities.

One of the most remarkable and the least understood of any of the assimilative and absorptive functions, is the ability shown by one part of the body to appropriate from the foods the elements necessary for its own rebuilding, while the same elements pass through other organs untouched. The body has the power, also, not only to make use of the foods, but to use up the blood tissue itself. Just how this is done is also a mystery.

There is surely a great lesson in industry here, and

one of the most profound studies in economics, physics, and chemistry.

Habitual worriers use up force and become thin more quickly than those whose work is muscular. Those who spend their lives fretting over existing conditions, or worrying over things which never happen, use up much brain force and create disagreeable conditions within, resulting in digestive ills. These again react on the body and continue the process of impoverishment of the tissues.

Certain it is that improper foods affect the disposition, retard the spiritual growth, and change the current of one's life and of the lives about one. Therefore the intelligent care of the body—the medium through which the soul communicates with material surroundings—is a Christian duty.

"The priest with liver trouble and the parishioner with indigestion, do not evidence that skilled Christian living so essential to the higher life."

Man has become so engrossed and hedged about with the complex demands of social, civic, and, domestic life, all of which call for undue energy and annoyance and lead him into careless or extravagant habits of eating and living, that he forgets to apply the intelligence which he puts into his business to the care of the machine which does the work. Yet the simple laws of nature in the care of the body are plainer and easier to follow than the complex habits which he forms.

The "simple life" embraces the habits of eating as well as the habits of doing and of thinking.

The whole problem of perfect health and efficient activity is in keeping the supply of assimilated food equal to the demand, in keeping a forceful circulation that the

*nourishment may freely reach all tissues and the waste
be eliminated, and in full breathing habits that sufficient
oxygen be supplied to put the waste in condition for
elimination.*

CONTENTS

CHAPTER I

PURPOSES OF FOOD

CHAPTER II

CLASSIFICATION OF FOOD ELEMENTS

CHAPTER III

CLASSIFICATION OF FOODS

CHAPTER IV

HEAT AND ENERGY

BEVERAGES AND APPETIZERS

Contents

Contents

ILLUSTRATIONS

What to Eat and When

THE purposes of food are:
To supply the material out of which the body may rebuild the tissues.

To produce heat, and to liberate muscular and mental energy.

Every particle of body substance is constantly changing. The new material for cells and tissues, the substance to supply the energy needed in the metabolic work of tearing down and rebuilding, the energy used in the digestive process of converting the food into condition to be assimilated, and the energy used in muscular, brain, and nerve movement must all be supplied by food.

Every effort of the brain in the process of thinking, every motion, and every muscular movement requires energy which the food must supply.

The body is composed of a vast number of cells varying according to the tissue or organ in which they are found. The characteristic of all living matter is that it constantly reproduces itself. Cells perform their appointed work, wear out, and must be replaced by new ones or derangements follow.

The new cells constantly being formed, increase in size and in so doing push the wornout, dying, and dead cells out of the way. The process of building and eliminating continues within the body and on its surface every instant of life.

An idea of the number of dead cells constantly being thrown off from every part of the body may be gained by noticing the amount of dead skin cast off. The fine scales of "scarf" or "dead" skin, which we easily rub off in a friction bath, are composed of these dead cells which have been crowded out by the hosts of vital cells constantly forming beneath. The process is the same in every tissue and organ. The dead or worn-out matter within the body is burned by oxygen and put in condition to be carried by the blood to the organs of elimination, the kidneys, intestines, lungs, and skin.

Much waste is eliminated in liquid form through the sweat glands. It is said that stokers throw off four pounds of water and waste a day through the skin.

In the growing child the process of building and of eliminating is active and rapid. In the youth it is less rapid, in the adult still less, but unless the process is kept active, stagnation and death ensue.

Daily exercise is necessary to keep up the body activities; yet very few take the trouble to secure daily a complete, thorough circulation of blood, especially through the vital organs and the deeper tissues. Perfect circulation is the key-note of health.

Activity of any kind necessitates the expenditure of energy. The process is a chemical one and in all chemical processes heat is necessary to cause the decomposition of elements and their recomposition into different substances.

Heat in its turn has two functions. It enables the chemical changes to be carried on which fit the food for the use of the various tissues, and it burns to an ash the wornout products of the body's activity, fitting them for elimination.

It keeps the tissues flexible and the secretions fluid; coagulation takes place when the secretions become cold.

As previously stated, food in the body, then, is needed for two purposes:

(1) to build and maintain the cell until its work is done;

(2) to furnish the heat necessary to decompose the food into its elements, and to produce the energy by which all the body processes are carried on.

That the food may be appropriated by the body it must be not only proper in kind and quantity, but the body must also be in condition to digest, absorb, and assimilate it and to eliminate the waste, otherwise the body needs are not met.

Food Elements

It is the nourishment which *the body assimilates and appropriates to its needs* which counts in food economy, *not necessarily the amount consumed.*

Therefore if the food is to economically serve its purpose, the body must be in a condition to digest and assimilate it—*this condition depends largely on perfect circulation, correct position of organs, and correct breathing habits.*

Of the fifteen to twenty substances contained in foods and comprised in the body, the principal ones are oxygen, hydrogen, carbon, nitrogen, chlorin, sodium, potassium, magnesium, iron, calcium, phosphorus, and sulphur. The differences in the forms of matter lie in the proportions in which these elements are combined.

Those containing the largest proportion of nitrogen are called *Nitrogenous* foods or *Protein*—such as meat, eggs, and some vegetables.

Those containing the largest proportion of carbon are known as *Carbonaceous*—such as cereals, sugar, and fat.

The four food elements, indispensable to life, either of plant or animal, are oxygen, hydrogen, carbon and nitrogen.

Carbon combined with oxygen forms carbon dioxid.

Oxygen, nitrogen, and carbon dioxid largely form the air.

Oxygen and hydrogen form water.

Calcium, iron, magnesium, sodium, and potassium are used in the formation of the various tissues and secretions of the body.

The substances contained in living organisms are the same as those in inorganic matter, only in different complexities as appropriated to the needs of each organism.

The difference between living and non-living matter is in the relative proportion and arrangement of the same elements.

Before it is fit to supply the needs of the body, the raw material must undergo a chemical change.

It has been demonstrated by scientific investigation that no unorganized elements, such as pure nitrogen, pure iron or magnesium, are assimilated by the system and converted into its various structures.

While the body needs carbon, it cannot use coal; it needs nitrogen, yet it cannot appropriate it to rebuilding bone and muscle, until, by chemical action with other elements, it has been converted into complex substances called proteins.

The muscles, ligaments, and labor-performing structures contain the largest amount of nitrogen.

The fat contains the largest amount of carbon.

The brain, the nerves, and the bones contain the largest proportion of phosphorus compounds.

Yet, while the brain contains phosphorus, and the tissues nitrogen, the brain cannot be built up by eating elementary phosphorus, nor the muscles by pure nitrogen, but compounds rich in phosphorus or nitrogen may be utilized.

Plants use the simple compounds of the earth, air, and soil, and, within their own cells, build them up into such complex substances as starch, sugar, protein, fat, and salts, putting them in condition for man and other animals to appropriate to their use.

All plant life is compounded from the elements in the soil, air, and water, by the action of the sun's rays. The rays of heat and light store something of their power in latent heat and energy in these plant compounds.

The end of plant life is the completion of its compounds—when it has matured them, the plant dies.

All organic matter is thus formed by the action of the sun's rays on inorganic matter.

The gluten of wheat is formed from the chemical union of nitrogen in the air and nitrogen in the soil with other substances.

The starch of wheat and other grains is from carbon

which the plant has taken from the soil and combined with other substances.

All meats are largely derived from plants which have appropriated the elements from the soil, water, and air. The chemical processes of the animal convert the energy latent in the plant food into the more concentrated form of meat. The animal thus performs a part of the chemical work for man—the digestive organs of one animal convert the food contained in certain plants, into a substance more easily assimilated by another animal.

Man would need to eat a large amount of nitrogen-containing plants in order to get as much protein as is contained in one egg or in a piece of lean meat the size of an egg. It is because the nitrogen is in such condensed form in meat and eggs that one is likely to take more than the system can handle, if he eats too freely of these two foods, particularly of meat. We will discuss this question more fully under "Proteins."

Most domestic animals take their food elements from air and water, as well as from the compounds which the plants have formed, while wild animals and some domestic ones, such as hogs and chickens, make use of meat as well.

The greater part of muscle, nerve, and gland is composed of *protein*.

When the muscles are exercised constantly they use up their protein and must have it resupplied, or the muscle substance will waste. When the muscles are exercised freely, as in the laborer, or the athlete, they need more building material.

The skeleton is composed largely of deposited *salts*, as *calcium*. If, therefore, the growing child be not supplied with a sufficient amount of this substance, the bones will be weak and liable to deformity and the teeth will be slow in coming or will be small and malformed. Children need foods rich in lime.

The elements which supply heat and keep up muscular activity are *starches, fats, and sugars.*

It must be apparent to every thoughtful person, that, since the nerves, muscles, and glands are composed largely of protein and the skeleton largely of calcium salts, in order to furnish the body with the elements necessary for growth and repair, all of these elements, as also the energy-producing substances, must be provided.

Each individual, therefore, should learn how much he requires to replace his daily waste, both for rebuilding tissue and for supplying heat and energy.

The day laborer, though he may do more muscular work than an athlete in training, expends scarcely any nervous energy. Therefore he needs less protein in his diet than one does who expends both nervous and muscular activity, as does the athlete.

CHAPTER II

CLASSIFICATION OF FOOD ELEMENTS

BY foodstuffs are meant the chemical elements appropriated by the animal for the use of the body, as previously described.

By foods are meant those articles of diet found in the market which contain the chemical elements used by the body in various combinations. Bread, for example, contains all of the foodstuffs and has been called the staff of life, because it sustains life. This refers to bread made from the whole of the grain. White bread, as commonly eaten, is not the "staff of life."

Foods may contain elements, not foodstuffs, and not used by the body, but cast out as waste. Certain foods, such as sugar, corn-starch, olive oil, and egg albumin, contain only one foodstuff, as will be noted in the following classification, in which the foodstuffs are grouped according to the body uses.

The classification of foods is based on the principal organic foodstuffs they contain. The preponderance of the elements in any one food determines its chief use in the body.

It will be remembered that the chief uses of foods are to produce heat and energy, to build the tissue of the growing child, and to repair the tissues in the child and the adult.

Nearly all foods are made up of a combination of substances.

The following tabulations give the classification of foods based on their predominating elements.

Nitrogenous foods:

>   Lean meat
>   Eggs
>   Gluten

Carbonaceous foods:

>   Sugars
>   Starches
>   Root and tuberous vegetables
>   Green vegetables
>   Fruits
>   Fats

Carbo-nitrogenous foods:

>   Cereals
>   Legumes
>   Nuts
>   Milk

Vegetables are mixtures of sugars and starches;

Fruits are mixtures of sugars, vegetable acids, and salts;

Milk, legumes, cereals, and nuts contain a more equal division of sugars, fats, and proteins, and are therefore represented as carbo-nitrogenous;

Lean meats, with the exception of shell-fish, contain no starch, but all meats contain protein, fat, and water.

Foodstuffs
- Inorganic { Water, Salts
- Organic
  - Carbonaceous (producing heat & energy)
    - Starches { Corn-Starch, Sago, Tapioca
    - Sugars { Glucose, Cane Sugar, Syrups, Honey
    - Fats { Lard, Olive Oil, Butter
  - Nitrogenous (for growth and repair)
    - Proteins { Egg Albumin, Gluten, Lean Meat

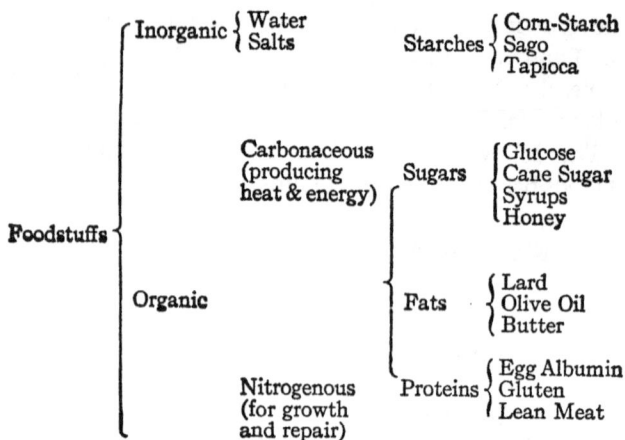

In the above tabulation, examples are given of foodstuffs which are almost pure representatives of their classes.

Corn-starch, sago, and tapioca are practically pure starch, containing very little of any other element;

Glucose, cane sugar, syrups, and honey are almost pure sugar;

Butter, lard, and olive oil are nearly all pure fat;

Egg albumin, gluten of flour, and lean meat are almost pure protein.

As previously stated, however, no food contains but one element of foodstuffs.

NITROGENOUS FOODSTUFFS OR PROTEINS

Protein is a complex combination consisting of seventeen elements. The digestive organs split up protein into these seventeen substances, and they enter the blood thus split. When they reach the tissues, each tissue selects the elements it needs and recombines them according to its own peculiar functional uses.

Meat and eggs contain the complete protein.

Protein exists in all vegetables, but few vegetables contain protein which is made up of the whole seventeen substances, hence more vegetable food has to be eaten to secure the protein in the quantity and combination necessary to maintain life.

Of these seventeen elements the predominating ones are nitrogen, sulphur, and phosphates. The predominance of nitrogen has given the proteins the name nitrogenous.

Proteins are the tissue builders.

In this connection it may be well to state that blood is a tissue; thus meat and eggs build the blood, as well as muscle and sinew.

All nitrogenous foods contain considerable carbon —mostly in the form of fat in the meat elements— but the carbonaceous foods contain so little protein that the protein elements do not appreciably enter into the nutrition.

Carbon and nitrogen in the carbo-nitrogenous foods are about equal in proportion.

The nitrogenous or protein elements in the body constitute about one-fifth of its weight. They form the basis of blood, lymph, muscle, sinew, bone, skin, cartilage, and other tissues.

Worn-out body tissue is constantly being torn down and eliminated and the protein in the foods must daily furnish material for repair, as well as for building new tissue.

A young animal's first need is for growth, as it has not learned to exercise sufficiently to use much latent energy. The first food it receives is an animal product—milk to babes and other mammals—while the young chicken or bird is nourished by the yolk of the egg contained within it. Sufficient yolk substance remains within the chick when it is hatched to sustain its life for the first day or two.

Nitrogenous foods are more concentrated and contain less waste; thus a smaller bulk is required than of vegetables and fruits. According to recent experiments, the average adult requires from two to four ounces of nitrogenous foods a day, to repair the waste. Happily, when more is consumed, the system has the power up to a certain limit (depending on the physical condition and the daily activity), to eliminate an excess.

It is needless to say that if the daily waste is not replaced, digestion and nutrition suffer. The system must have the two to four ounces necessary to supply the nitrogen daily excreted, or the tissues themselves wll be consumed.

The proteins, of which meat is the principal member, are classified as:

Albuminoids: albumin (white of eggs), casein (curd of milk), myosin (the basis of lean meat and gluten of wheat);

Gelatinoids: (connective tissue of meat);

Extractives: (appetizing and flavoring elements).

If protein material is taken into the body in excess of its needs the excess is used as fuel. While vastly more expensive, an excess of protein is worth no more as fuel than starch is; 1 gram of protein produces 4.1 calories of heat, no more than 1 gram of starch.

The proteins produce heat and energy when the supply of sugars, starches, and fats is exhausted, but proteins alone form muscle and the larger part of blood and sinew.   They are, in this sense, the most important of foods; they are also the most costly.

An excess of protein, usually eaten in the daily intake of food, then, is of no practical use and can be eliminated with great benefit to the pocketbook. Meat once a day is sufficient.   The excessive consumption of meat can be lessened with no lack of nutrition to the body.   The trouble is that meat is the first thing thought of for a meal; it is easily prepared and housewives are not willing to use the thought and effort necessary to secure a balanced meal without it.

CARBONACEOUS FOODSTUFFS

The carbonaceous foods are those used by the body for heat and energy and are so named because they contain a large proportion of carbon—the heat-producing element.

It is the carbon in wood, which, uniting with oxygen, produces heat and light.

The carbonaceous foods are all composed of carbon, hydrogen, and oxygen, the difference between them being in the different proportions in which these elements are combined.

They are divided into two classes, Carbohydrates and Fats.

The carbohydrates embrace the *sugars* and *starches* and include such substance as **Carbohydrates** the starches of vegetables and grains (notably corn, rice, wheat, and the root vegetables), and the sugar of milk, of fruits, vegetables, and the sap of trees.   Their chief office is to create energy.

The starches are converted into sugar, so they are together given the one name of carbohydrate. The name means that carbon and hydrogen are contained in them in such a proportion that when oxygen unites with the hydrogen, water is produced and the carbon is liberated. In this chemical process heat is produced. One gram of carbohydrate produces 4.1 calories of heat.

They are almost entirely absent from meat and eggs, the animal having converted them into fats.

When the digestive organs are in a normal condition carbohydrates are easily digested.[1] They do not play a large part in the growth of the body tissues, but they are utilized by the body to spare the consumption of the fat which is stored in the tissues as a reserve. This explains their action in preserving but not producing fat. When there is an excess of fat and the desire is to reduce, the carbohydrates should be limited that the body may call on the reserve fat for heat and energy.

Few realize that after the starches and fats have been consumed in heat and energy the tissues are consumed.

The assimilation of the carbohydrates is almost complete, so that the energy derived from them may be closely calculated.

SUGAR

There are many varieties of sugar. Those commonly used as foods are, cane sugar (sucrose), fruit

[1] For the process of digestion and the action of the digestive juices on the various food elements, see *Let's Be Healthy*, by Susanna Cocroft.

sugar (levulose), sugar of milk (lactose), sugar of malt (maltose), sugar of grapes or corn (glucose), maple sugar, honey, and saccharin—a coal-tar product. They are derived from plants, from trees, and from tubers or other vegetables.

Cane sugar (sucrose) is derived from the juice of the sugar cane and from beets. One-third of the world's supply of sugar is derived from the sugar cane and two-thirds from beets.   From two to ten per cent. of sucrose may be obtained from the maple tree. It is also found in the sugar pea.

All sugars are carbohydrates—carbon, hydrogen, and oxygen—the oxygen and hydrogen being in the proportions which form water (two atoms of hydrogen and one of oxygen).

Brown sugar is granulated sugar in an early stage of refinement.

Maple sugar is obtained by boiling down the sap of the maple tree.   It is often adulterated with other sugars or with glucose from corn, because they are cheaper.   This adulteration does not make it unwholesome, but causes it to lose its distinct maple taste.

The nutritive value of sugar is said to be about ninety-five per cent.

Glucose was formerly derived almost entirely from grapes.   Later the process was discovered by which the starch in corn was converted into glucose.   It is produced so much more cheaply from corn that this is now the chief source of supply.

Glucose is also found in most of the fruits, in combination with other sugars.   It needs little change to be absorbed by the system and quickly overloads the digestive apparatus if much of it is eaten.

It is pure, wholesome, and cheap, and for this reason it is often combined with other sugars. It is not so sweet as cane sugar, though just as nutritious. Many of the syrups on the market are made from it.

Candy is often made from glucose instead of from molasses or cane sugar.

Much candy, unless one is actively exercising, tends to produce indigestion.

While glucose is wholesome, it ferments readily.

Before sugar can be used by the system, it is changed into the easily absorbed form of the sugar in grapes, by a ferment in the small intestine. Hence digested sugar in the body is called grape sugar.

Milk sugar needs less chemical change than other sugars and is taken almost at once into the circulation. It is contained in the natural food for the infant.

The digested sugar (grape sugar) is further changed in the body into glycogen. When an excess of sugar or starch is consumed, it is stored within the body as glycogen, until required.

Sugar is perhaps a better food than starch, because less force is required for its digestion and it is easily assimilated, being more readily converted into dextrose than are starches.[1] Moreover it furnishes the heat and energy needed by those having small power to digest starch.

Sugar is soon oxidized, and, for this reason may be eaten by those who need to use an extra amount of muscular strength, or to get strength quickly. It yields heat and energy within thirty minutes after

[1] PUBLISHER'S NOTE: The conversion in the body of starch and sugar into grape sugar, then into dextrose, then into glycogen, the glycogen being again broken up into grape sugar, is fully explained in Susanna Cocroft's book *Let's Be Healthy*.

eating, and in times of great exertion or exhausting labor, the rapidity with which it is assimilated gives it advantage over starch. Because it is so quickly converted into energy it is valuable for children at active play.

Experiments with soldiers on forced marches, and in Arctic explorations, have shown the value of sugar as a food, in enabling the men to withstand hunger, thirst, and fatigue. Taken in excess, however, particularly by those of sedentary habits, it clogs the system as does ˙ny other excess of material, creating difficulties for the liver and kidneys.

During muscular activity, four times as much sugar is consumed in the body as is ordinarily used in the body processes.

Used in limited quantities, therefore, according to the muscular or brain power exercised, sugar is one of the best foods for the production of energy.

When much sugar is eaten the starches and fats in the food should be lessened to avoid overloading the system.

When eaten in excess, sugar may temporarily appear in the urine unaltered.

It might be inferred that, as all starch must be converted to sugar before it can be used by the body, starches might be discarded and replaced by sugars. A small quantity of sugar, however, soon surfeits the appetite, and if the foods were confined to those having a surplus of sugars, sufficient food would not be eaten to supply other needs of the body. This lack of appetite occasioned by an excess of sugar is due, partly, to the fact that the gastric juice is not secreted so freely when there is much sugar in the stomach.

2

Because of the slower secretion of gastric juice and the surfeit of the appetite occasioned by them, sweetened foods should not be used at the beginning of a meal, and, while a moderate amount of sugar is desirable, a surfeit will cause indigestion. This is particularly liable when one eats sufficient starch and sugar at a meal and then eats candy between meals.

Sugar is so readily oxidized and supplies heat and energy so promptly, that the fats stored in the tissues are not called on until the latent energy in the sugar is used. The power of sugar to fatten thus lies in sparing the use of body fat; when starch and fat are used in addition to sugar an excess of fat quickly results. Therefore, those who wish to reduce in flesh should eat sparingly of sugar that the starches and fats may be used to furnish energy, but sugar should be as freely used as the system can handle it, by those who wish to build up in flesh.

Broadly speaking, about one-fourth of a pound of sugar, daily, in connection with other foods, is well utilized by the system, the quantity depending on whether one leads an active or a sedentary life.

The natural flavor of fruits and grains is very largely destroyed by sugar, which is used too freely on many articles of diet. Sugar should never be added to fruits while cooking, if intended for immediate use, as the acids of the fruits neutralize a portion of the sugar. More sugar is thus used than is needed after the cooking process is completed.

The sweet taste in all fruits and vegetables is due to the presence of sugar. Sweet potatoes, beets, carrots, parsnips, turnips, grapes, figs, and dates are especially rich in sugar, and when these are furnished with a meal, in any appreciable quantity, the starches should be restricted—notably bread, Irish potatoes, and rice.

Those who do hard work in the open air, because of the increased oxidation, can consume larger quantities of sugar in pie or other pastry, which ordinarily would be difficult to digest. One who lives an indoor life should refrain from an undue indulgence in such foods.

For one who is undernourished, sugar is a desirable food, if the starch be diminished in proportion as the amount of sugar is increased; but the tendency in sweetening foods is to take more starch also than the system requires, since it is the carbohydrate foods which are ordinarily sweetened—not the proteins.

On account of their latent heat and energy, sugars are more desirable in cold weather than in warm. For this reason Nature supplies them more abundantly in the root vegetables, eaten more freely in cold weather. More puddings and heavier desserts may be eaten in cold weather.

The desire of the child for sweets is a natural one, because the child uses much energy, and sugar supplies this energy with less tax of the digestive system. When the child begins to eat more solid foods, if sugar is used in abundance for sweetening, he is no longer attracted by the mild sweetness of fresh milk, and it is well not to sweeten cereals or other foods, also to limit other sweets, when the child turns against milk, in order to restore the taste for this valuable food. Many authorities state that a child, up to its third year, should not be allowed to taste artificial sweets, in order that the appetite may not be perverted from the natural sweets of milk.

Sugar is better supplied the child in a lump or in

home-made molasses candy, rather than in the sweetening of porridge, oatmeal, or bread and milk, etc.

Molasses is readily absorbed and is mildly laxative,
and when young children are not allowed to eat too
much, it assists in keeping the bowels open.

Sweet fruits, fully ripened, contain much sugar
and should be freely given to the child.

Starch   Starch is one of the most important
carbohydrates. It is formed from the
carbon dioxid and water in the air and in the soil by
the chemical action of the sun's rays on the cells of
living plants.

As stated, corn-starch, sago, tapioca, and arrowroot
are practically pure starch. Rice is almost pure
starch.

Corn-starch is obtained from young maturing corn;
tapioca comes from a tropical plant, cassava; sago
from the pith of the sago palm; arrowroot from a
plant of the same name, a native of the West Indies.

Starch lacks flavor and for this reason all starchy
foods are seasoned with salt. Salt increases the
activity of the saliva and pancreatic juices.

All starches must undergo much chemical change
by action of the saliva and the intestinal juices, before
they can be used by the body.

The digestion is begun by the saliva in the mouth
and is continued in the stomach, by the saliva, until
the gastric secretions begin to act.

Starch is not acted on by the gastric juice but passes
unchanged into the intestines, where it is converted,
by the pancreatic juice, into dextrin, maltose, and
glucose. It is thus absorbed into the blood.

After the digested starch passes into the blood it is

taken to the liver and is there changed into glycogen and is stored in reserve. When the system needs to produce energy it is first furnished by the glycogen. When this is exhausted the fats and proteins are used.

The *starches* and *sugars* then are really the energy "reserves" of the body, any excess over the daily needs being stored until required.

Starchy foods should not be given to any one in whom, from disease or derangement, the starch-converting ferments, ptyalin in the saliva and pancreatin in the pancreatic juice, are lacking.

Because the child has not developed the ferment in sufficient quantities necessary for starch digestion, starchy food must not be given to a child under twelve to eighteen months; at least not until he has teeth and chews his food. Then he should be given starchy food in the form of a crust or hard cracker which he chews thoroughly and mixes with saliva.

Potatoes or bananas which the child does not masticate, should not be given him under the age of two years.

Fat is the most concentrated form of fuel **Fat** and is readily oxidized. It has about twice the fuel value of carbohydrates. It is almost pure carbon, hence less chemical work is required to convert it into fuel, but more oxygen is needed.

The average fat person does not breathe deeply and does not take in sufficient oxygen to cause a combustion of the fat and produce energy. He is thus inclined to be lethargic.

A pound of fat has about three times as much fuel value as a pound of wheat flour, which consists largely of starch.

Common examples of fat are butter, cream, the

fat of meat and of nuts, and the oil of grains and seeds
—notably the cocoanut, olive, and oatmeal.

Fat forms about twenty per rent. of the weight of
the normal body.

The body cannot remain in health for long unless a
proper amount of fatty food is eaten. Muscular and
nerve action, and the formation of the digestive secretions are all dependent on the energy derived from
the combustion of fat. Its use in this way spares the
tissues from destruction in the chemical processes
necessary to life.

Both carbohydrates and fats are composed of carbon, hydrogen, and oxygen, the difference being that
there is less oxygen in fat. One pound of starch requires one and one fifth pounds of oxygen for perfect
combustion, while one pound of suet requires three
pounds of oxygen. One ounce of fat yields two
and one-half times as much energy as an ounce of
sugar or starch.

Fats are not digested in the stomach. The connective tissue about the fat is dissolved here, and the
fat is passed on into the small intestine, where it is
acted on by the bile and the intestinal juices. These
first change the fat into an emulsion and then into
the form of soap and glycerin. In this saponified
form, it is in condition to be absorbed and carried to
the tissues, where it is assimilated and used in energy.
The commercial production of soap from oil is similar
to the chemical change in the body of fat into soap.

The supply of fat stored in the body depends on the
quantity consumed with the food, on the quantity
used up in heat and energy in muscular or mental
exercise. The quantity assimilated depends somewhat on the condition of the nerves. If the nerves

are weak, they do not strongly direct digestion and assimilation and less fat is used in the digestive and assimilative processes; thus, in case of weak nerves more fat is often stored in the tissues. An excess of fat often indicates sluggish nerve activity.

Manual laborers require more fat for energy than do people whose habits are sedentary. School-children, or children who play hard, should have sufficient fat and sugar.

Butter and Cream. The fat present in milk, depends of course, on the quality of the milk. There is as much butter-fat in a glass of fresh Jersey milk as in a glass of cream from the milk of some cows. The cream from some Jersey cows is eighty per cent. butter-fat.

Skimmed milk contains very little fat. If milk is drunk by the adult, as a means of storing up more fat within the body, the cream, if assimilated, should be stirred into it.

The Fat of Meat. This should be thoroughly cooked. All meats in the process of baking or frying should be covered, in order to retain the moisture. The fat in well-roasted beef is nutritious, but *to make fat easily digestible it should be well masticated so as to break up the tissue fibers which surround it.*

While fried foods are difficult of digestion (see page 192) because the surface albumin is coagulated and the hot fat forms a coating around it, making it difficult for the digestive juices to reach the tissue, the fat of bacon is more easily dissolved because of the delicacy of the fibers surrounding the fat cells. If thinly sliced and fully immersed in its own grease in the process of frying, bacon is an easily digested fat.

The process of smoking the bacon renders it easier of digestion.

Cooked bone-marrow is an easily digested form of fat which is usually relished by those to whom any other fat is repulsive. It is useful in some forms of anemia, as it contains considerable iron.

Eels, salmon, and mackerel contain much fat.

The Eskimos extensively use both whale and seal oil as a food.

The yolks of eggs are also rich in fat.

Cod-Liver Oil, pressed from the liver of the codfish, is easily absorbed and assimilated by some. The odor is not pleasant and a little lemon juice, salt, baking soda, or any flavoring substance may be added to make it palatable. The pure oil taken in this way is, perhaps, preferable to the prepared emulsions.

Olive Oil is derived from ripe olives. It is often used when cod-liver oil is not well borne. Many take olive oil for the purpose of rounding out the figure with fat. If the system will assimilate fat, taken in quantities, the fat may be stored; but, as a rule, one is underweight because of a failure to assimilate the regular diet and overloading the digestive organs with fat will not cause a better assimilation. If the lack of flesh is due to sluggish assimilation exercise should always accompany a diet for the building of flesh.

Olive oil, in moderation, is a good food when much heat and energy are required, but if one's occupation is sedentary, much fat is not necessary.

Cotton-seed Oil is often substituted or mixed with the cheaper grades of olive oil. It is wholesome, if fresh, but has not the pleasing flavor of the olive.

Nut Oils are good, but, with the exception of peanut

butter, are not often used. English walnuts, hickory nuts, pecans, cocoanuts, and Brazil nuts contain much oil. Nut oils are not well borne by some, hence nuts must be sparingly used by them. If taken they should be used with salt, and be thoroughly masticated.

Almond oil and olive oil are used in cooking, to some extent.

To summarize—digested sugar is called dextrose or glucose; digested starch becomes first dextrin, then maltose (animal sugar); digested protein is peptone; and digested fat is saponified fat.

WATER

No food element is more important for the needs of the body than water. It is composed of oxygen and hydrogen. It forms the large part of the blood and lymph.

The body will subsist for weeks on the food stored in its tissues; it will even consume the tissues themselves, but it would soon burn itself up without water, and the thirst after a few days without it almost drives one insane.

Though it produces force only indirectly, it is entitled to be classed as a food, because it composes about two-thirds of the weight of the body and a large part of all the tissues and secretions. Yeo estimates that the supply of water to the body should be averaged at half an ounce for each pound of body weight.

It has been estimated that from four to five pints of water are excreted each day by the body and therefore a similar amount should be consumed daily.

The average individual at normal exercise, requires about seventy one and one half ounces of water daily, which equals about nine glasses (one glass of water weighs one-half pound). Some of this may be obtained from the food.

By reference to Tables I to V it will be noted that water forms a large percentage of all food, particularly of green vegetables and fruits.

In order that the body may do efficient work in digestion and in the distribution of the nutrient elements of the foods, and that the evaporation from the body may be maintained, the water in the foods, together with the beverages drunk, should consist of about seventy-five per cent. liquid to twenty-five per cent. nutrient elements, or about three times as much in weight as proteins, fats, and carbohydrates combined.

Much of the water taken passes through the system without chemical change and is constantly being thrown off by the skin, lungs, kidneys, and intestines.

Some of the water is split up into hydrogen and oxygen to unite with other substances in the chemical changes carried on during the process of digestion, and some water is obtained from the food by the union of hydrogen and oxygen liberated by the action of the digestive juices.

Few people give much thought to its resupply; yet, ignorant of the cause, they suffer from its loss, in imperfect digestion and assimilation, and in kidney and intestinal difficulties. If it is withheld from the diet for a while, marked changes occur in the structure and processes of the body. The effect is seen in the lessening of the secretions, the increasing dryness of all the tissues, including the nerves, and if the lack is long continued, in progressive emaciation, weakness, and death.

Water is the heat regulator of the body, and the more energy used, either in work or in play which results in more heat and evaporation, the more water is required. An animal, if warm, immediately seeks water.

It is constantly being used in the body to form solutions in which the waste products are held so that the eliminative organs may dispose of them.

It is the chief agent in increasing the peristaltic action of both the stomach and intestines, thus aiding in mixing the food with the digestive juices and assisting the movement along the alimentary canal.

It increases the flow of saliva and of the digestive juices and aids these juices in reaching every particle of food.

It dissolves the foods, and helps in the distribution of food materials throughout the body, carrying them in the blood and the lymph from the digestive organs to the tissues, where they are assimilated.

The blood carries the water to the various secreting and excreting glands and its increased pressure aids both the secreting and excreting activity. The digestive organs secrete their juices more freely, digestion is aided, more nutriment is rendered absorbable, more carbon dioxid is liberated, and more oxygen is taken into the blood which thereby is made richer and more life-giving.

One engrossed in business or household cares may forget to take water between meals. In such a case, the blood, in order to preserve its volume, must draw the water from the tissues, which, in consequence, become less moist. The mouth becomes dry, saliva is scanty, appetite fails, the digestion is not so active, the digestive and other secretions are lessened in quantity, the food in process of digestion becomes more solid, its absorption in the intestine is more difficult, it moves slowly along the intestinal canal, and constipation results. The body is not so well nourished and falls a more ready prey to disease.

The supply of fluid furnished to the kidneys is not sufficient, the urine becomes more concentrated and irritation may result. The foundation is thus laid for derangements of the kidney function.

To maintain the equilibrium of the body forces, water drinking should be established as a permanent habit and be firmly adhered to as a part of the daily program.

Many claim that one's thirst, as in the desire for food, is the only safe guide to the amount and time of drinking, but these desires are largely matters of habit, and tastes are often perverted. Unless the condition is abnormal or the mind becomes so intensely active that one fails to listen to the call of Nature, *the system calls for what it has been in the habit of receiving* and at the stated times it has been in the habit of receiving it. It does not always call for what is good for it.

Plants thrive after a shower because the falling water brings down the impurities in the air which constitute plant food. Rain-water for household use, therefore, should never be collected during the early part of a shower or rain storm.

Spring water, from its filtration through earth rich in mineral deposits, usually contains a certain percentage of those minerals, as salt, sulphur, or iron, dissolved through the action of the carbon dioxid contained in the water. Some of these springs have become famous health resorts.   The contained carbon dioxid gives spring water its pleasant, sparkling taste. Spring water is remarkably free from organic life.

Water as used in cities usually needs careful filtration and purification to rid it of its contained sand and other impurities.   The housewife whose water supply is derived from rivers does this on a small scale when she strains out the mud and sand from the water which she is often compelled to use when the river is in flood and full of impurities.

Drinking water should be perfectly clear and without odor.   Even a small amount of decomposing vegetable or animal matter can be detected by its odor, if the water is confined for a short time in a bottle or closed jar.

The health of the body depends to a large degree on the purity of the water.   Contaminated water is a menace to health.

Water which appears perfectly clear may be badly contaminated with typhoid or other germs.   For this reason no water should be used until it has been boiled if one is not sure of its purity.   Water from wells near barns and cesspools is often impure.

"Hard" water, as derived from wells, is usually rich in calcium and magnesium.   When water contains a large percentage of these substances, it usually causes constipation and indigestion and may aid in the formation of gall-stones or gravel.

The kidneys are especially the great eliminators of water and aid in maintaining the equilibrium of the blood.   Except in conditions in which they need rest, water should be freely drunk in order to stimulate them to activity and to assist them in throwing off the body waste held in solution.

One cannot form a better habit than that of drinking two or three glasses of water on first arising and then exercising the stomach and intestines by a series of movements which alternately contract and relax the walls of those organs, causing their thorough cleansing.

This internal bath is as necessary as the cleansing of the skin. Often, in gastritis or a catarrhal condition of the stomach, a large amount of mucus will collect in the stomach over night, and the cleansing of the mucous lining of the digestive tract is then most important.

If in good health, two or three glasses of cool water, vigorous exercises for the vital organs, and deep breathing of pure air, followed by a cold bath, will do more to keep the health, vigor, clear skin, and sparkling eye than fortunes spent on seeking new climates, mineral waters, or tonics.

When cool water in the morning seems to chill one, a glass of hot water may be followed by a glass of cool.

The free drinking of water aids the activity of the skin, keeping the tissues moist and the glands active.

Effervescing waters are usually drunk for their cooling and refreshing effect. They should not be drunk to excess as they are usually combined with syrups or sugar and will thus occasion derangement of digestion, flatulence, and in some cases palpitation from the excess of gas which presses on the diaphragm and impedes the action of the heart.

Mineral waters are drunk for the action of the salts which they contain and are used for their laxative or their medicinal effect. Kissengen, Hunyadi Janos, Epsom, Carlsbad, and our own Saratoga are examples of laxative waters. These all contain sodium and magnesium sulphates and are known as "bitter" waters.

Table waters, as Apollinaris, Vichy, or others containing carbon dioxid are refreshing and wholesome and may be used in nausea and vomiting for their quieting effect. Those who are unable to take milk will often find its digestion will be aided if the milk be mixed with Vichy or seltzer water.

When water is used as a hot drink it should be freshly drawn, brought to a boil, and used at once. This sterilizes it and develops a better flavor.

Cold water should be thoroughly cooled, but not iced. Water is best cooled by placing the receptacle on ice rather than by putting ice in the water. Impure or contaminated ice will contaminate water.

The theory has long been held that water drinking at meals is injurious, the objection being that the food is not so thoroughly masticated if washed down with water, and that it dilutes the digestive juices. But this theory is now rejected by the best authorities.

When water drinking at meals is allowed to interfere with mastication and is used to wash down the food, the objection is well taken, but one need rarely drink while food is in the mouth; the water should be taken at rest periods between mouthfuls.

Thorough mastication and a consequent free mixing of the food with saliva is one of the most essential steps in digestion, and the flow of gastric juice, as the flow of saliva, is stimulated by the water.

It is singular that the use of water at meals has long been considered unwise when the free use of milk, which is about seven-eighths water, has been recommended.

The copious drinking of cool water from a half hour

to an hour before a meal will cleanse the stomach and incite the flow of saliva and gastric juice, thus aiding digestion.

Moreover, the digestive cells secrete their juices more freely and the sucking villi absorb more readily when the stomach and intestines are moderately full, either of food or water, and to fill the stomach with food requires too much digestive and eliminative activity.

Water taken before meals passes through the stomach before the food, washes away any mucus that may have collected over the mouths of the gastric glands, stimulates them to activity, and prepares the stomach to receive the food.

Results obtained, in building up about twenty thousand thin women, show that the free drinking of liquid at meals has a tendency to increase flesh. Probably one reason for this is the cleanliness and greater freedom it gives to the absorbing and secreting cells of the mucous lining of the digestive tract, the stronger peristalsis it occasions, and the consequent better digestion.

When one wishes to reduce in flesh, water drinking at meals is restricted.

If the contents of the stomach have become too concentrated or solid, the water will render it more liquid, hence will aid the admixture with the gastric juices and will enable it more readily to pass the pyloric orifice.

Drinking at meals, therefore, has many more arguments in its favor than against it.

All who have a tendency to the deposit of uric acid in the tissues, as in gout, should drink freely of water to lessen the deposit of salts from the blood which must maintain its proportion of fluid.

More water should be drunk if the meal consists largely of protein. The nitrogen it contains is eliminated in a short time by the kidneys, the amount of urine is increased, and more water must be drunk to make up the loss.

In sickness, as in fever, the increased respiration causes a corresponding loss of water from the skin and the lungs. If the bowels are active as in diarrhea, much water is lost in this way. The increase in the heat of the body also tends to dry all the secretions, hence water must be taken to keep them in proper fluidity.

The patient is often too ill to ask for water or will forget to ask for it. Constipation may result from this cause. It must be a part of the nurse's duty to see that a sufficient amount is taken. An excess of cold water, if hastily taken, may cause cramps. If slowly sipped it will do no harm.

Water may be given in fever in the form of lemonade; a small pinch of soda will make it effervescent and more refreshing.

There is no tonic like water, exercise, and fresh air. The safe method is not to allow the habit of drinking water with regularity to be broken, unless for some necessary purpose, and then the habit should be reinstated as soon as possible.

Soft water, that is, water containing no lime or other mineral, is best. Hard water which causes any degree of curdling of soap, or a lime crust in the bottom of a teakettle, renders digestion difficult.

Bacteria are killed and much of the mineral matter is deposited by boiling the water. Boiled water tastes flat or insipid. It may regain its original, fresh taste by filling a jar half full of water, and shaking the jar so that the air passes through the water.

SALTS

The salts of sodium, potassium, magnesium, calcium and some other substances, are necessary for proper bodily functioning. Taken with the food, they pass into the tissues without change and can be recovered, unchanged, from the tissues and the urine.

The uses of some of these substances are not thoroughly understood, but if deprived of them, the nutrition of the body suffers.

Lime (calcium) is necessary for the bones and teeth and to preserve the coagulability of the blood.

Sodium chlorid (common salt) aids the formation of hydrochloric acid and the activity of the pancreatic juice.

The salts of iron are necessary for the blood.

Other salts are also needed to carry on the chemical reactions in the digestive system.

Cereals, all vegetables, fruits, and nuts furnish both calcium salts and sodium, potassium, and magnesium, which are the salts in the blood and lymph. Minerals are also abundant in dried legumes (beans and peas).

Fruits and nuts contain the least amount of these salts, and meats, vegetables, and cereals follow in the order named, cereals, that is the whole of the grain—not the white flour—containing the most. Any diet, therefore, which recommends the use of fruits and nuts to the exclusion of other foods, depletes the system of some of the body-building elements. The system may seem to thrive for a time on such food because, perhaps, of the rest given to overworked organs, but eventually the body lack will manifest itself; anemia may appear or malnutrition become evident.

Milk furnishes salts in proper proportion for building the bones and teeth of the baby; because of the lime which it contains it is a good food for the growing child. After the child is one year old, eggs may be added to the diet. During the first year the albumin and fats in the egg are not well digested. It is especially essential that children be furnished milk and eggs that they may be assured of the proper proportion and quantity of calcium salts for growth.

Sodium chlorid (common salt) has been for ages recognized as an important element in food, so important that in Eastern countries it is the symbol of hospitality and friendship.

When taken in moderate quantities, salt increases the activity of the gastric secretion and aids the appetite. When taken in excess, as many who have formed the salt-eating habit do, it is an irritant to the mucous membrane of the stomach and intestines and may interfere with nutrition, causing dyspepsia, gastroenteritis or diarrhea from the continued irritation.

The habit indulged by some of nibbling at salted nuts of various kinds, at and between meals, may for a short time satisfy the needs of the body for more salt than is usually taken with the food, but such a habit persisted in will cause acidity of the stomach from overstimulation of the hydrochloric acid producing glands; it will also decrease the fluidity of the blood by causing the water to be drawn from the blood for the use of the tissues. Irritative action is also exerted on the kidney, as any excess of salt is excreted by this organ. For this reason salt is often prohibited for those suffering from any inflammation of the kidney, in Bright's disease, etc.

When chemical tests show an excess of hydrochloric acid, salt should be omitted from the diet.

A diet consisting largely of vegetables needs the addition of sodium chlorid to supply sufficient salt for body uses; likewise more salt than is contained in grass and fodder is needed for animals, particularly for those producing milk. The scientific farmer salts his cattle regularly, while wild animals travel miles and form beaten paths to springs containing salt.

In rectal feeding, it is known that food absorbs more readily through the large intestine if salted. It is probable that salt, in normal proportions, also aids absorption in the stomach and small intestine.

Potassium is next in importance to sodium as it constitutes the chief salt in the muscles. It also aids the action of the digestive secretions and the maintenance of the reaction of the urine. Potatoes and apples are valuable foods on account of the potassium they contain.

Calcium, if in excess, may cause the formation of calculi, renal or biliary. It is also found in the tartar which accumulates on the teeth, in the hardening walls of the arteries in arteriosclerosis, etc. All of the cabbage family are rich in calcium. Many mineral waters and the water from many wells contain it in excess.

Those addicted to gall-stones, gravel, etc., should particularly avoid "hard" water.

Phosphorus and sulphur are obtained by the body from eggs and milk and from such vegetables as corn, cauliflower, asparagus, and turnips.

Iron is necessary in forming the pigment of the red blood corpuscles.

If, through some disturbance in digestion, absorption or assimilation, the iron taken in the food is not utilized, or is insufficient in amount, the blood-making organs do not receive the necessary amount of this substance and the red corpuscles are not formed in sufficient numbers. The blood becomes poor in hemoglobin, and the individual becomes pale and loses vitality. This condition is known as anemia.

CHAPTER III

CLASSIFICATION OF FOODS

IN the previous chapters, we have given the classification of the elements in foods (foodstuffs) which supply the body needs. In this chapter the foods commonly used are classified according to the predominance of these elements.

CARBONACEOUS FOODS

While all foods contain a combination of elements, some contain a greater proportion of carbohydrates and fats, and are classed as *carbonaceous*.

Of the carbohydrates, next in importance to the sugars and to the starches in their purest form **Roots and Tubers** (cornstarch, tapioca, sago, and arrowroot), come the roots and tubers, such as potatoes, sweet potatoes, beets, parsnips, turnips, and onions.

The following table shows the proportion of various foodstuffs in these vegetables. The skins of the vegetables are included.

38

TABLE I

Roots and Tubers

FOOD MATERIALS	Water per cent.	Protein per cent.	Fat per cent.	Carbo-hydrates per cent.	Ash per cent.	Food Value per pound Calories
Sweet Potatoes	69.4	1.5	0.3	26.2	2.6	440
White Potatoes	75.0	2.1	0.2	22.0	0.7	295
Parsnips	64.4	1.3	0.4	10.8	1.1	230
Onions	86.0	1.9	0.1	11.3	0.7	225
Beets	87.0	1.4	0.1	7.3	0.7	160
Carrots	88.2	1.1	0.4	8.2	6.0	210
Turnips	92.7	0.9	0.1	0.1	0.6	120

Potatoes. It will be noted from the table given above that sweet potatoes contain a larger percentage of carbohydrates, hence they produce more heat and energy than any other vegetable; next to the sweet potato comes the Irish or white potato.

While the white potato contains two per cent. of protein, this is almost all located in a very thin layer immediately beneath the skin, so that when the potato is peeled in the ordinary way, the protein is removed. This is true of many vegetables. They lose their distinctive flavor, as well as their value as tissue-building foods, when the skins are removed, especially before cooking. Many vegetables may be peeled after being cooked and their value in nutrition is thus increased. All tubers gain in dietetic value if they are cooked in their skins, the thin outer covering being removed after the cooking process is completed. The ordinary cook, however, is unwilling to take the trouble to prepare them in this way.

In vegetables as usually prepared for the table the proportion of carbohydrates is increased and the proportion of protein is diminished. The skins render many of the foods unsightly, hence they are discarded in the preparation for cooking.

When a potato is baked the outer skin is readily separated from the less perceptible layer containing the protein. Potatoes boiled in their skins retain the protein.

In the white potato, of the twenty-two per cent. of carbohydrates, three and two-tenths per cent. is sugar and eighteen and eight-tenths per cent. is starch. In the sweet potato ten and two-tenths per cent. is sugar and sixteen per cent. is starch.

Since sugar digests more quickly than starch, the sweet potato digests more quickly than the white. Because of the large percentage of carbohydrates in each, it is a mistake to eat these two vegetables at the same meal, unless the quantity of each is lessened. For the same reason, bread and potatoes, or rice and potatoes, should not be eaten to any extent at the same meal, unless by one who is doing heavy manual labor, requiring much energy.

Onions. Only about four per cent. of the onion represents nourishment; the eleven and three-tenths per cent. of carbohydrates is made up of two and eight-tenths per cent. sugar and the rest of extractives. Of the extractives the volatile oil, which causes the eyes to water when onions are peeled, is the most important.

The onion is not, therefore, so important for its actual nourishing qualities as for its relish and flavor, and for this it is to be commended.

It is a diuretic, encouraging a free action of the

kidneys. Because of its diuretic value it is commonly called a healthful food. An onion and lettuce sandwich stimulates the action of the kidneys and is a nerve sedative.

The volatile oil makes the raw onion difficult for some to digest and, in that case, should be omitted from the diet.

Beets. There is no starch in beets, their seven and three-tenths per cent. of carbohydrates being sugar. They possess, therefore, more nutritive value than onions, and they are easily digested. It will be noted that it takes many beets to make a pound of sugar.

There are no more delicate or nutritious greens than the stem and leaf of the beet. These greens contain much iron and are valuable aids in building up the iron in the blood, thus aiding in the correction of anemia.

Carrots. Carrots are valuable as food chiefly on account of their sugar. They are somewhat more difficult of digestion than beets and they contain more waste. They make a good side dish, boiled and served with butter or cream.

Turnips. Turnips have little value as a food. Their nutriment is in the sugar they contain. For those who enjoy the flavor they are a relish, serving as an appetizer, and, like the onion, are to be recommended as a side dish for this purpose.

Parsnips. Like carrots, parsnips are chiefly valuable for their sugar and for the extractives which act as appetizers.

Since turnips, carrots, onions, and parsnips owe a part of their nutritive value to the extractives which whet the appetite for other foods, it follows that, if one does not enjoy their flavor or their odor, these vegetables lose in value to that individual as a food. If one does enjoy the flavor, it adds to their food value, therefore *taste for the flavors of all foods should be cultivated.*

Green Vegetables   The question may be asked with reason: "Why do we eat green vegetables?" They contain only about four per cent. nutriment, as will be seen in Table II, and are mostly made up of water and pulp. It will be noted that they are distinctly lacking in protein and in carbohydrates; hence, they have little food value.

Some of them, however, contain acids which tend to increase the alkalinity of the blood, and salts which are needed by the system.

Their merit lies in the fact that they have distinct flavors and thus whet the appetite. Another reason why green vegetables are thoroughly enjoyed is because they come in the spring, when the appetite is a little surfeited with the winter foods.

They are diuretic, helping the kidneys and the skin to rid the system of waste.

Because of their bulk of waste they are useful in constipation as they act as a stimulus to the peristaltic action of the bowels; thus they are more laxative to the intestines than the root vegetables, partly because of the salts which they contain and partly because of the undigested vegetable fiber. This vegetable fiber, being coarse, assists in cleansing the mucous lining of the stomach and intestines. They are diuretic and, if for no other reason than for this cleansing of the kidneys, and to make the stomach and intestines more efficient, the use of green vegetables is to be commended, and it is well to eat freely of them.

TABLE II

GREEN VEGETABLES

FOOD MATERIALS	Water per cent.	Nitrogenous Matter per cent.	Fat per cent.	Carbohydrates per cent.	Mineral Matter per cent.	Cellulose per cent.	Fuel Value per pound Calories
Cabbage	89.6	1.80	0.4	5.8	1.3	1.1	165
Spinach	90.6	2.50	0.5	3.8	1.7	0.9	120
Vegetable Marrow	94.8	0.06	0.2	2.6	0.5	1.3	120
Tomatoes	91.9	1.30	0.2	5.0	0.7	1.1	105
Lettuce	94.1	1.40	0.4	2.6	1.0	0.5	105
Celery	93.4	1.40	0.1	3.8	0.9	0.9	85
Rhubarb	94.6	0.70	0.7	2.3	0.6	1.1	105
Water Cress	93.1	0.70	0.5	8.7	1.3	0.1	110
Cucumbers	95.9	0.8)	0.1	2.1	0.4	0.5	10
Asparagus	91.7	2.20	0.2	2.9	0.9	2.1	110
BrusselsSprouts	93.7	1.50	0.1	3.4	1.3	0.4	95
Beans (string)	8.92	2.3	0.3	7.4	0.8	7.0	·195
Beans (dried)	12.6	22.5	1.8	59.6	3.5	0.0	1605
Peas (green, shelled)	74.6	7.0	0.5	16.9	1.0	0.0	465

In larger cities, fresh vegetables are in the markets the year around, but if they are raised in greenhouses, or in any way forced, they lack the flavor which comes with natural maturity and they also lack the full amount of iron given by the rays of the sun. If raised in the south and shipped from a distance, they are not fresh and they do not have as good an effect on the system as when fresh and fully matured by the sun.

Greens, as spinach, chard, dandelions, and beet tops,

as previously stated, contain iron and build red blood corpuscles.

Cabbage, of which there are many varieties, contains much sulphur. If fermentation exists in the intestines the sulphur unites with hydrogen causing gas of an unpleasant odor.

They promote the formation of calcium oxalate in the urine and should be avoided as a food by any one inclined to gout, rheumatism, or gall-stones.

Cabbage is usually not well digested by invalids.

Eaten raw, because of its bulk, it is laxative. Some dyspeptics, who cannot digest cooked cabbage, digest raw cabbage readily.

Celery is wholesome when cooked, because of the milk and butter in which it is prepared. Eaten raw the fiber is hard for the digestive juices to dissolve and should be thoroughly masticated. It has little nutritive value save for its appetizing flavor.

Because of the salts, largely sulphates and phosphates, which it contains, celery has been called a nerve food, but the proportion of these is so small that their food value is negligible.

Tomatoes are easily digested and are refreshing, They are not well borne by some and on account of the oxalic acid they contain should not be used by those having an excess of uric acid.

Asparagus, because of its delicate flavor and appearance early in spring, is a vegetable universally liked. It is easily digested and may be eaten by invalids; they usually greatly relish it. Its particular food value lies in its sulphur and in its value as an appetizer.

Rhubarb is one of the most wholesome of vegetables and is being much more widely used. Thoroughly cooked it is digestible and a natural laxative.

Its tart flavor and appearance in early spring render it a pleasant change from the ordinary diet. Eaten in excess, like cabbage, it produces calcium oxalate in the urine and should not be eaten in large amounts by those inclined to gout.

All fresh vegetables should be masticated to almost a fluid consistency; otherwise, they are difficult of digestion, containing, as they do, so much fiber.

Fruits

Technically speaking, fruits include all plant products which bear or contain a seed. They are valuable for their acids and organic salts—citrates, malates, or tartrates of potassium, sodium, magnesium, and calcium.

They are composed for the most part of starch, sugar, water, and various organic acids, cellulose, and pectin. (Pectin is the substance which jellies under heat.) Fruits which do not contain pectin must be combined with others which do, or with gelatin, if jelly from them is desired.

The organic acids in fruits are readily split up in the body, and form alkalis. For this reason acid fruits are useful in certain acid conditions of the stomach, because they combine with the stomach acids, liberating substances which cause an alkaline reaction.

The citrus fruits—oranges, lemons, grapefruit and limes—are rich in citric acid.

Malic acid is found in gooseberries, peaches, pears, apples, currants, and apricots.

Tartaric acid is prominent in grapes.

The value of fruits as a food depends largely on the amount of starch and sugar they contain, though their agreeable odor and taste, by furnishing variety in the diet, render them, also, of great value as appetizers.

As a rule they contain too much water to be of great food value if eaten alone.

The organic acids and salts contained in fruits are of value as they stimulate the activity of the kidneys and lessen the acidity of the urine. The urine may even be rendered alkaline by them; hence, when a test shows evidence of too much uric acid, acid fruits are used to neutralize the acids in the tissues, particularly the acids of the citrus fruits.

The fruit juices are readily absorbed and the potassium calcium, sodium, and magnesium they contain are liberated with the formation of alkaline carbonates.

These alkalis are largely eliminated through the kidneys, which accounts for the diuretic effect of fruits, their acids and salts stimulating the activity of the kidneys.

The seeds in the small fruits are not digested, but they serve the purpose of increasing intestinal peristalsis and of assisting the movement of the contents of the intestines. The skin and the fiber of fruits also assist the intestines in this way, just as the fiber in vegetables does.

All acid fruits—particularly lemons, limes, grapefruit, and oranges—stimulate the action of the skin as well as the kidneys and whenever the kidneys and skin are not sufficiently active, these fruits should be eaten freely.

In case of an excess of hydrochloric acid in the stomach, lemon juice or citrus fruits are valuable about half an hour *before* a meal, as when taken on an empty stomach they decrease the secretion of hydrochloric acid.

When the secretion of hydrochloric acid is limited, acids are given *after* a meal to supplement the deficiency, or stimulate the glands to activity.

Sweet or *bland* fruits are those containing a lesser percentage of acids. Among these are pears, raspberries, grapes, bananas, blackberries, blueberries, melons, and some peaches, apples, and plums.

Of this class of fruits, dates, figs, prunes, and grapes (raisins), furnish most nutriment, because, as will be noted by Table III, these fruits contain a large amount of carbohydrates in the form of sugar.

The protein in these sweet fruits is largely in the seeds and, as the seeds are not digested, they have no real food value for the individual.

Figs and prunes, peaches, apples, and berries are laxative—probably the laxative action of figs and berries is due to the seeds, and of the others to the salts and acids they contain, and to the cellulose or fibrous material which furnishes bulk.

TABLE III

FRUITS

FOOD MATERIALS	Water per cent.	Protein per cent.	Ether Extract per cent.	Carbo-hydrates per cent.	Ash per cent.	Cellulose per cent.	Acids per cent.
Apples	82.50	0.40	0.5	12.5	0.4	2.7	1.0
Apricots	85.00	1.10	0.6	12.4	0.5	3.1	1.0
Peaches	88.80	0.50	0.2	5.8	0.6	3.4	0.7
Plums	78.40	1.00	0.2	14.8	0.5	4.3	1.0
Cherries	84.00	0.80	0.8	10.0	0.6	3.8	1.0
Gooseberries	86.00	0.40	0.8	8.9	0.5	2.7	1.5

FOOD MATERIALS	Water per cent.	Protein per cent.	Ether Extract per cent.	Carbo-hydrates per cent.	Ash per cent.	Cellulose per cent.	Acids per cent.
Currants	85.20	0.40	0.8	7.9	0.5	4.6	1.4
Strawberries	89.10	1.00	0.5	6.3	0.7	2.2	1.0
Whortleberries	76.30	0.70	3.0	5.8	0.4	12.2	1.6
Cranberries	86.50	0.50	0.7	3.9	0.2	6.2	2.2
Oranges	86.70	0.90	0.6	8.7	0.6	1.5	1.8
Lemons	89.3	1.00	0.9	8.3	0.5	1.5	1.8
Pineapples	89.3	0.04	0.3	9.7	0.3	1.5	7.0
Pears	83.90	0.40	0.6	11.5	0.4	3.1	0.1
Blackberries	88.90	0.90	2.1	2.3	0.6	5.2	1.6
Raspberries	84.40	1.00	2.1	5.2	0.6	7.4	1.4
Mulberries	84.70	0.30	0.7	11.4	0.6	0.9	1.8
Grapes	79.00	1.00	1.0	15.5	0.5	2.5	0.5
Watermelons	92.90	0.30	0.1	6.5	0.2	1.0	0.5
Bananas	74.00	1.50	0.7	22.9	0.9	0.2	0.5
Dates, dried	2.08	4.40	2.1	65.1	1.5	5.5	7.0
Figs, dried	2.00	5.50	0.9	62.8	2.3	7.3	1.2
Prunes, dried	2.64	2.40	0.8	66.2	1.5	7.3	2.7
Raisins	10.60	2.50	4.7	74.7	3.1	1.7	2.7

The astringent and acid taste of unripe fruits is due to the tannin and the acids. Oxygen is necessary to ripen fruits and the slow natural maturing of the fruit on the tree enables the oxygen to enter into combination with these substances, lessening their reaction and altering the starch into glucose or levulose.

Fruits ripened artificially lack this cnemical action of sun and oxygen, hence the decreased palatability and digestibility of fruits so ripened. If underripe fruits are freely eaten they ferment in the alimentary tract and this fermentation causes the colic, vomiting, and diarrhea so often experienced. Overripe fruit, from the decomposition products which have already begun to form and which are further released in the stomach or bowels, may produce the same results.

Care should therefore be exercised to select thoroughly ripe fruits which have not begun to decay.

In order to reach their destination in fair condition, outwardly, many fruits are picked before they are ripe. Bananas are commonly picked green, because they decay so quickly that if they were picked ripe they would spoil before reaching the northern markets.

One test of a naturally ripened apple is to cut it with a steel knife—if the blade turns black, or if the cut surface of the apple turns brown in a few minutes, it should not be eaten, for it indicates an excess of tannin. It is this tannin which gives the small boy excruciating pains from his green apples.

It will be recalled that the tannin from the bark of trees toughens the skin of animals and forms leather. The effect on the membrane of the stomach and intestines, from the tannin in food, is not so pronounced, because of the activity and resistance of living matter.

The juice of lemons and oranges is most valuable in seasickness and scurvy, and is of benefit in nausea. A slice of lemon will often clear a coated tongue and give a refreshing sense of cleanliness to the mouth, especially in feverish conditions. Sour lemonade is one of the best drinks in summer because of its thirst-allaying qualities.

Table III shows that *bananas* contain nearly twenty-three per cent. of carbohydrates, which, in an immature state, are largely starches. The natural ripening

4

process changes the starch to sugar, thus making them more easily digested. The starch globules, when not matured on the tree, are not easily broken and are thus difficult of digestion.

Bananas should not be given to children under two years of age because before this age the ptyalin and pancreatin are not sufficiently developed to digest the starch.

Many of the inhabitants of the tropics use bananas almost to the exclusion of other food and appear well nourished. They obtain them from the tree when the fruit has thoroughly ripened, the starch having been transformed by Nature into an easily digested product.

The reason many find they cannot digest bananas, as purchased in our markets, is due to the fact that the fruit is immature and unripe.

The banana meal or flour is usually thoroughly digestible, is nourishing, and has an agreeable taste. Invalids can often take banana meal in the form of gruel; it makes an appreciated addition to a limited diet. Made into a porridge and eaten with cream it is valuable in conditions of inflammation of the gastro-intestinal tract. The addition of a few drops of lemon juice renders it palatable to those who like an acid flavor. Children enjoy it as a variation from cereals. It is relished by typhoid fever patients as a change from milk.

It must be carefully cooked and well prepared as, like oatmeal, it can be spoiled by insufficient or poor cooking. Owing to the limited demand it is not obtainable in all markets, as it has not yet become popularized.

Grapes, because of their wholesome qualities, are

useful to the system, as they contain sodium, iron, magnesium, potassium, and calcium. Because of their appetizing flavor they are universally enjoyed, and because they are cheap are universally used. The skins and seeds are indigestible and, if swallowed, may cause severe irritation or obstruction of the intestines. Grapes are rich in sugar, and on this account must not be eaten by diabetics.

Grape juice, when unfermented, is a valuable drink, in health, or for the convalescent. It is agreeable in taste and is mildly laxative. Added to other fruit juices, as lemon or orange, it allays thirst and furnishes a pleasant flavor, but on account of its high percentage of sugar does not allay thirst when used alone.

Apples, so universally used, are easily digestible when ripe, and may be prepared in so many ways that they constitute a valuable addition to the diet. Their laxative qualities, when taken on an empty stomach, as before breakfast, or just before retiring, are well known. They are thus valuable in constipation, and in some forms of dyspepsia may, with benefit, be eaten raw.

Apples should be thoroughly masticated.

The apple peel contains potassium salts and should be eaten with the fruit.

Most invalids digest apples better if they are cooked, especially baked. Stewed apples may have the beaten white of eggs whipped into them and invalids who revolt against eggs can take them thus prepared.

Because of the sugar necessary in cooking them they should be avoided by diabetics, and in conditions in which there is irritation of the gastro-intestinal tract.

Quinces are indigestible when raw, but well baked and eaten with cream are appetizing and nourishing.

Pineapples, if thoroughly ripe, contain a ferment which will digest protein, rapidly softening and disintegrating the tissue of meat. Like the pancreatic ferment it acts in both alkaline and acid mediums. Pineapple juice, therefore, is exceedingly valuable as an addition to the diet. The coarse fibers also have a laxative action. Care must be taken, however, to use this fruit only when it is well ripened, as when green, it is indigestible.

The juice of pineapple, because of the action of the ferment in dissolving tissue, is valuable in many forms of sore throat, particularly when accompanied by an ulcerous condition. The effort should be made to hold it in the mouth, allowing it to trickle down the throat by degrees.

Dried fruits are less palatable than fresh. Many of them, as prunes and raisins, are nourishing, but others, as citron, are indigestible, and should be finely chopped if used as flavoring.

Dried or evaporated fruits, through the action of heat, either artificial or from the rays of the sun, have lost the water they contained, and are preserved by their own sugar.

Dried grapes, or raisins, because of their sugar, soon satiate the appetite if eaten raw, but if cooked or added to cereals, puddings, or breads, enhance the palatability and nourishing qualities of these foods.

Dates and figs used in the same way, in cereals or puddings, are equally valuable.

Dried currants are the most indigestible of the

dried fruits, owing to their large amount of skin in proportion to the nutriment.

NITROGENOUS FOODS

As previously stated, in a mixed diet, meat and eggs are the chief sources of nitrogenous foods. Next to these come the legumes.

Meat is composed largely of muscle fiber and contains connective tissue and fat. It has been estimated that beef contains one-third nutritive material, the other two-thirds being water and bone. Fat meat contains less nitrogenous material and less water than lean meat.

Meat

Lean meat is almost entirely digested in the stomach by the gastric juice, which changes it into peptone. It is needless to say that it should be thoroughly masticated, that the gastric juice may promptly act on it. If any part passes into the intestine undigested, the process is continued by the trypsin of the pancreatic juice.

The peptone is absorbed and carried by the blood and lymph to all tissues of the body, where it is used for growth and repair. As stated under "Heat and Energy," any excess of protein above that needed for growth and repair is oxidized if sufficient oxygen is breathed, yielding energy and heat, and the waste is eliminated through the kidneys and the bile.

For purposes of comparison, one pound of beef has been said to equal in nutritive value, two and one-half pints or five glasses of milk, one-half pound (two-thirds of an ordinary baker's loaf) of bread, and three eggs. However, these values vary.

TABLE IV

ANIMAL FOODS

FOOD MATERIALS	Water per cent.	Protein per cent.	Fat per cent.	Carbo-hydrates per cent.	Ash per cent.	Fuel Value per pound Calories
Beef, Fresh	54.0	17.0	19.0	....	0.7	1105
Flank	54.0	17.0	19.0	....	0.7	1105
Porterhouse	52.4	19.1	17.9	....	0.8	1100
Sirloin steak	54.0	16.5	16.1	....	0.9	975
Round	60.7	19.0	12.8	....	1.0	890
Rump	45.0	13.8	20.2	....	0.7	1090
Corned beef	49.2	14.3	23.8	....	4.6	1245
Veal:						
Leg cutlets	68.3	20.1	7.5	....	1.0	695
Fore quarter	54.2	15.1	6.0	....	0.7	535
Mutton:						
Leg, hind	51.2	15.1	14.7	....	0.8	890
Loin chops	42.0	13.5	28.3	....	0.7	1415
Lamb	49.2	15.6	16.3	....	0.85	967
Ham:						
Loin chops	41.8	13.4	24.2	....	0.8	1245
Ham, smoked	34.8	14.2	33.4	....	4.2	1635
Sausage:						
Frankfurter	57.2	19.6	18.6	1.1	3.4	1155
Poultry:						
Fowls	47.1	13.7	12.3	....	0.7	765
Goose	38.5	13.4	29.8	....	0.7	1475
Turkey	42.4	16.1	18.4	....	0.8	1060
Animal Viscera:						
Liver (sheep)	61.2	23.1	9.0	5.0	....	....
Sweetbreads	70.9	16.8	12.1	....	1.6	....
Tongue, smoked and salted	35.7	24.3	31.6	....	8.5	....
Brain:	80.6	8.8	9.3	....	1.1	....
Fresh Fish:						
Bass large-mouthed Black, dressed	41.9	10.3	0.5	....	0.6	215
Cod steaks	72.4	16.9	0.5	....	1.0	335
Shad roe	71.2	23.4	3.8	....	1.6	595
Whitefish, dressed	46.1	10.2	1.3	....	0.7	245

FOOD MATERIALS	Water per cent.	Protein per cent.	Fat per cent.	Carbo-hydrates per cent.	Ash per cent.	Fuel Value per pound Calories
Preserved Fish:						
Halibut, salted,						
smoked and dried	46.0	19.1	14.0	....	1.9	945
Sardines, canned	53.6	24.0	12.1	....	5.3	955
Salmon, canned	59.3	19.3	15.3	....	1.2	1005
Mollusks:						
Oysters, solid	88.3	6.1	1.4	3.3	0.9	235
Round clams re-						
moved from shell	80.8	10.6	1.1	5.1	2.3	340
Mussels	42.7	4.4	0.5	2.1	1.0	140
Crustaceans:						
Lobster, in shell	31.1	5.5	0.7	....	0.6	130
Crab, in shell	34.1	7.3	0.9	0.5	1.4	185
Shrimp, canned	70.8	25.4	1.0	0.2	2.6	520
Terrapin, turtle, etc.	17.4	4.2	0.7	...	0.2	105

The amount of fat in meat varies from two to forty per cent., according to the animal and to its condition at the time of killing.

The best meats are from young animals which have been kept fat and have not been subjected to any work to toughen the muscles.

It is possible to combine the fat and the lean of meat so as to meet the requirements of the body without waste. About ninety-seven per cent. of meat is assimilated by the system, while a large part of the vegetable matter consumed is excreted as refuse.

The compounds contained in animal foods are much like those of the body, therefore they require comparatively little digestion to prepare them for assimilation—this work having been done by the animal—while the vegetable compounds require much change

by the digestive system before they can be used in
the body.

The proportion of *albuminoids*, *gelatinoids*, and
extractives in meat vary with different meats and with
different cuts of the same meat.

The *albuminoids* of meat include the meat tissue,
or the muscle cells. These constitute by far the
greater part of the meat.

The *gelatinoids* are derived from the connective
tissue forming the sheath of the muscle and of bundles
of muscles, the skin, tendons, and the casing of bone.
Gelatins are made from these and, if pure and prepared in a cleanly manner, they are wholesome.

Gelatin is distinguishable in rich meat soups, which
jelly when cool.

The gelatinoids alone have not a large nutritive
value; they serve to spare the albumin from being
used, though they cannot replace albumin in the diet.
They also, to some extent, keep the muscles from being
consumed when starches, sugars, and fats are lacking.

The *extractives* are found most abundantly in the
flesh of animals and birds noted for their muscular
activity, as in game. Some of them exert a stimulant
action on the nervous system and others are appetizers, giving to cooked meats, broths, etc., their pleasing
flavor. In case of anemia, in which it is necessary to
build red blood corpuscles, the blood of beef, the
thought of which is usually repellent, may be made
very palatable if it is heated sufficiently to bring out
the flavor of the extractives, and then seasoned.

Unless the beef extracts on the market contain the
blood tissue, in addition to the extractives, they are
not particularly nourishing and are only valuable in
soups, etc., as appetizers.

Soups for nourishment should be made by cooking the bones, connective tissue, and a part of the meat. Bones and connective tissue alone make an appetizing soup, but it contains little nutriment.

One reason why meat soups should constitute the first course at dinner is because the extractives stimulate the appetite and start the flow of gastric juices. Bouillons contain no nourishment, but they may be used as stimulant restoratives to the muscles, or as a basis for vegetables, rice, or barley to give them flavor.

Roasted flesh seems to be more completely digested than boiled meat; raw meat is more easily digested than cooked; rare meat is more easily digested than that thoroughly cooked.

Roasted young chicken and veal are tender, easily masticated, and easily and rapidly digested in the stomach. This is one reason why the white meats are considered a good diet for the invalid, though veal is usually avoided in cases of dyspepsia, as, if too young, it may cause diarrhea; if too old, it is less digestible than beef.

Fat meats remain in the stomach a much longer time than lean meats; thus, gastric digestion of pork, which usually contains much fat, is especially difficult, requiring from three and one-half to four hours (see page 22).

Preserved and canned meats should be eaten with the utmost caution, care being taken to know that they are put up by firms which use extreme care in their preparation. Inferior meat is sometimes used in the preparation of these foods. If meats are not fresh and the canning not carefully done, they may become putrid after being put up.

Fish and *sea foods* are, many of them, rich in protein, as noted in Table IV.   They should never be used unless absolutely fresh.

The idea is prevalent that fish is a brain food.   Fish is easily digested and builds brain as well as other tissue, but no more readily than beef does, or any easily digested, absorbed and assimilated food which contains a goodly proportion of protein.

Lobsters are difficult of digestion and contain little nutrition, so are not valuable as a food, though they are relished by many on account of their flavor.

Oysters, raw, are easier to digest than when cooked. Oysters should not be eaten during the spawning season from May to September.

Mussels are nutritious when well prepared and are rapidly gaining in popularity.

Clams furnish a valuable and nutritious food when prepared in chowder form.   Clam broth will often be retained on an irritable stomach when other food is rejected by it.

Care should be taken to ascertain the method of their production as typhoid fever has been contracted from eating shell fish whose feeding beds were near or in polluted water.

Eggs   Eggs are excellent articles of food for nutrition and for tissue building.   They have practically the same value in the diet as meat, and make a very good substitute for meat.   Egg yolk in abundance is often prescribed when it is necessary to supply a very nutritious and easily as-similated diet.

Eggs consist chiefly of two nutrients—protein and fat (ten per cent.).   Because they contain so large a proportion of protein they are classified as nitrogenous foods.

The yolk, which is about one-third fat, contains iron, sulphur, potassium, calcium, magnesium, and phosphorus. The white contains some fat and phosphorus. The white and the yolk contain equal quantities of protein. The white of the egg is almost pure albumin.

The dark stain made by eggs on silver is due to the sulphur.

The iron in the yolk is a valuable assistant in building red blood corpuscles.

Eggs, in common with other proteins, are changed, mostly in the stomach, into peptone. That not digested in the stomach, as is the case with other proteins, is changed in the intestine.

If the egg is old, or if its absorption is delayed in the intestine, it decomposes, producing gas, and may cause intestinal disorder. For this reason no stale egg should ever be served, especially to an invalid.

One reason why eggs disagree with some is because too much fat is eaten at the same time. Egg yolk contains fat and if much extra fat is eaten indigestion and fermentation in the intestine may result. This is particularly true in those who digest fat with difficulty.

When eggs seem to disagree or the system does not assimilate them well on account of the fat in the yolk, and eggs are desirable to supply the protein in the diet, the whites, which contain practically no fat, may be used. They should be well beaten and if digestion is weak they may be mixed with fruit juices.

The citric acid in lemons and oranges partially

digests the egg, the gastric juice quickly changing it to peptone.

One method of preparing eggs, which is especially valuable for those having delicate stomachs, is in egg lemonade or orangeade. Thoroughly beat the egg, add the juice of half a lemon or orange, sugar to taste, and fill the glass with water.

Grape juice, cream, and cocoa, if assimilated, may be used in place of lemon or orange, in order to give variety when it is necessary to use eggs freely.

Eggnog is another means of taking raw eggs.

One method of testing the freshness of eggs is to drop them into a strong, salt brine made by adding two ounces of salt to a pint of water. A fresh egg will at once sink to the bottom. If the egg is three days old the surface of the shell will be even with the surface of the water and an egg two weeks old will float mostly above the surface.

The opinion is prevalent that a hard-boiled egg is difficult of digestion, but this depends entirely on the mastication. If it is masticated so that it is a pulp before being swallowed, a hard-boiled egg is readily digested.

A soft-boiled egg should not be boiled longer than three or four minutes, or better, should be put into warm water, be allowed to come to a boil, then set off the fire and the egg be allowed to remain in the water for ten minutes. This method cooks the egg through more evenly.

Another method of cooking the yolk evenly with the white is to put the egg in cold water, let the water come to a boil, and again immerse the egg in cold water. The immersing in cold water after boiling makes hard-boiled eggs peel readily.

CARBO-NITROGENOUS FOODS

Under this class come cereals, legumes, nuts, milk, and milk products. In these foods the nitrogenous and carbonaceous elements are more evenly proportioned than in either the carbonaceous or nitrogenous groups. The different food elements in this group are so evenly divided that one could live for a considerable length of time on any one food. Some animals build flesh from nuts alone, while the herbivorous animals live on cereals and plants.

Under cereals, used by man for food, come wheat, oats, rye, barley, rice, and corn. As· **Cereals** will be noted by Table V, cereals contain a large proportion of starch and are therefore used largely for heat and energy. Rice contains the largest proportion and next to rice, wheat flour.

TABLE V

CEREALS

FOOD MATERIALS	Water per cent.	Protein per cent.	Fat per cent.	Carbohydrates		Ash per cent.
				Starch, etc. per cent.	Crude Fiber per cent.	
Wheat	10.4	12.1	2.1	71.6	1.8	1.9
Rice	12.4	7.4	0.4	79.2	0.2	0.4
Oats	11.0	11.8	5.0	59.7	9.5	3.0
Rye	11.6	10.6	1.7	72.0	1.7	1.9
Breads and Crackers:						
Wheat bread	32.5	8.8	1.9	55.8	....	1.0
Graham bread	34.2	9.5	1.4	53.3	....	1.6
Rye bread	30.0	3.4	0.5	59.7	....	1.4

| | Water per cent. | Protein per cent. | Fat per cent. | Carbohydrates | | Ash per cent. |
FOOD MATERIALS				Starch, etc. per cent.	Crude Fiber per cent.	
Soda crackers	8.0	10.3	9.4	70.5	....	1.8
Graham crackers	5.0	9.8	13.5	69.7	....	2.0
Oatmeal crackers	4.9	10.4	13.7	69.6	....	1.4
Oyster crackers	3.8	11.3	4.8	77.5	....	2.6
Macaroni	13.1	9.0	0.3	76.8	....	0.8
Flours and Meals:						
Flour, wheat	12.5	11.0	1.0	74.9	....	0.5
Corn Meal	15.0	9.2	3.8	70.6	....	1.4
Oatmeal	7.6	15.1	7.1	68.2	....	2.0

The values as given in the table refer to the whole of the grain. When the outer coverings are removed, as in the white flour and the outer covering of rice, the proportion of carbohydrates is increased and the protein and ash are almost entirely eliminated.

There is no part of the world, except the Arctic regions, where cereals are not extensively cultivated. From the oats and rye of the north, to the rice of the hot countries, grains of some kind are staple foods.

An idea of the importance of cereal foods in the diet may be gathered from the following data, based on the results obtained in dietary studies with a large number of American families: Vegetable foods, including flour, bread, and other cereal products, furnished 55 per cent. of the total food, 39 per cent. of the protein, 8 per cent. of the fat, and 95 per cent. of the carbohydrates of the diet. The amounts which cereal foods alone supplied were 22 per cent. of the total food, 31 per cent. of the protein, 7 per cent. of the fat and 55 per cent. of the total carbohydrates— that is, about three-quarters of the vegetable protein, one-half of the carbohydrates, and seven-eighths of the vegetable fat were supplied by the cereals. Oat, rice, and wheat breakfast foods

together furnished about 2 per cent. of the total food in protein,
1 per cent. of the total fat, and 4 per cent. of the carbohydrates
of the ordinary mixed diet, as shown by the statistics cited.
These percentage values are not high in themselves, but it must
be remembered that they represent large quantities when we
consider the food consumed by a family in a year.[1]

If one's work calls for extreme muscular exertion,
the cereals may be eaten freely, but if one's habits
are sedentary, and the cereals are used in excess, there
is danger of clogging the system with too much starch.
Indeed, for one whose occupation is indoors and requires little muscular activity, a very little cereal
food, such as bread, cake, etc., will suffice; the carbohydrates will be supplied, in sufficient quantity,
in vegetables.

Mineral matter is supplied in sufficient quantity
in almost all classes of foods.

Cereals and legumes supply nutrients at less price
than any class of foods; therefore a vegetarian diet
involves less expense than the mixed diet. An entirely vegetarian diet, however, gradually induces
a condition of muscular weakness in many people,
resulting in a loss of strength. A well-proportioned
mixed diet is best to give strength and activity of both
body and mind.

Meat, eggs, and milk, which usually supply the
proteins, are the most expensive foods, and when
these, for any cause, are eliminated, a large proportion
of proteins should be supplied by the legumes.

Perhaps no food is as commonly used as **Wheat**
wheat in its various forms. It is composed of:

[1] Charles D. Woods, Dr. Sc., in *Cereal Breakfast Foods.*

1. The nitrogenous or protein compound, chiefly represented in the cerealin and the gluten of the bran. This is removed from white flour and from much of the so-called "whole wheat" flour.

2. The starch—the center or white part of the kernel.

3. The fats, occurring chiefly in the germ of the grain.

4. The phosphorus compounds, iron, and lime, found in the bran.

The kernel of wheat consists of the bran or covering, which surrounds the white, pulpy mass of starch within. In the lower end of the kernel is the germ.

Flour. In the old-time process of making flour the wheat was crushed between stones and then sifted, first, through a sieve, which separated the outer shell of the bran; then through bolting cloth, which separated the white pulp from the inner bran coating. It was not ground as fine as in the present process, thus the gluten, phosphorus, and iron (all valuable substances) were, in the old process, nearly all left out of the white flour. The second bran coating, left by the second sifting, was not so coarse as the outer shell but coarser than the inner. Care was not formerly observed in having the grain clean before grinding, the bran containing chaff and dirt, so that it was not used as food but was considered valuable for stock, and was called "middlings."

In the modern process of crushing the wheat between steel rollers, the white flour of to-day contains more of the protein from the inner coat of the bran than the white flour of the old process; hence, it is more nutritious.

Bran. Objection is sometimes made to bran because the cellulose shell is not digested, but bran contains much protein and mineral matter and even though it is crude fiber, as previously stated, this fiber has a value as a cleanser for the lining of the stomach and intestines, and for increasing peristalsis, thus encouraging the flow of digestive juices and the elimination of waste. In bread or breakfast foods, it is desirable to retain it for its laxative effect.

Bran has three coats—the tough, glossy outside, within this a coat containing most of the coloring matter, and a third coat, containing a special kind of protein, known as cerealin. The two outer layers contain phosphorus compounds, lime, and iron. All three coats contain gluten.

Gluten flour is made of the gluten of wheat. It is a valuable, easily digested food, containing a large proportion of protein and little starch. Gluten bread is used by those who wish to reduce in flesh and in diabetic cases.

Whole wheat flour does not contain the whole of the wheat, as the name implies; it, however, does contain all the proteins of the endosperm and the gluten and oil of the germ, together with all of the starch. As a flour, therefore, it is a more balanced food than the white flour, because it contains more nitrogenous elements.

Graham flour is made from the entire wheat kernel with the exception of the outermost scale of the bran. It contains the starch, gluten phosphorus compounds, iron, and lime. It is the most desirable of the flours because, containing the bran, it assists in digestion and elimination, and the phosphorus, iron, and lime, are valuable body builders.

Nutri meal is much the same as Graham flour, the

5

chief difference being that the bran is ground finer. The wheat is ground between hot rollers, the heat bringing out the nutty flavor of the bran. Bread made from it is not only nutritious, but delicious in flavor. It contains all of the nutrition of the wheat.

Bread. As must be implied from the foregoing, the nutri meal, or graham flours are necessary for bread if it is to be used as a complete food, the "staff of life." The white bread is made from flour which is almost pure starch; the lime, phosphorus compounds, and iron are removed.

Perhaps no form of prepared food has been longer in vogue than bread. It has been known since history began. When the entire wheat kernel is used it probably maintains and supports life and strength better than any single food, but bread is not the "staff of life" unless the entire kernel is in the flour.

Children should be given Graham bread or Graham crackers containing the whole of the grain in order to obtain the balanced food and the nutritive materials which are not obtained in bread made of white flour. Lime for the teeth and the growing bones is in the bran.

The more porous the bread the more easily it digests. When full of pores, it is more readily mixed with the digestive juices.

The pores in bread are produced by the effort of the gas, released by the yeast, to escape. When mixed with water, the flour forms a tenacious body which, when warm, expands under the pressure of the gas from the yeast, until the dough is full of gas-filled holes. The walls of gluten do not allow the gas to escape, and thus the dough is made light and porous. The more gluten the flour holds, the more water the dough will take up and the greater will be the yield of bread; hence, the more gluten, the more valuable the flour. If the bread is not porous, the fermentation is not complete, and the bread is heavy.

The albumin in the walls of the expanding bubbles causes substances which contain beaten eggs to be more porous when baked.

Yeast is a plant fungus. In its feeding, the plant consumes sugar, changing it into alcohol and carbon dioxid. If the bread contains no sugar the yeast plant will change the starch in the flour into sugar for its feeding.

Many housewives, realizing that the bread begins to "rise" quicker if it contains sugar, put a little into the sponge. Unless a large quantity of sugar is put in, the yeast will consume it and the bread will not have an unduly sweet taste.

As the yeast causes fermentation, alcohol forms in the dough. This is driven off in the baking. If the bread is not thoroughly baked, fermentation continues and the bread turns sour.

Bread is not thoroughly baked until fermentation ceases. It is claimed that fermentation does not entirely cease with one baking; this is the basis of the theory, held by some, that bread should be twice baked. The average housekeeper bakes an ordinary loaf one hour.

Time must be given for the products of fermentation to evaporate, during the cooling of the bread, before it is eaten.

Hot or insufficiently cooked bread is difficult of digestion, because it becomes more or less soggy on entering the mouth and the stomach, and the saliva and gastric juices cannot so readily mix with it.

The best flour for bread is that made from the spring wheat, grown in cooler climates, because it is richer in gluten than the winter wheat. The winter wheat flour is used more for cakes and pastries.

Bread made with milk, is, of course, richer and more nutritious than that made with water, and bread made with potato water contains more starch; both of these retain their moisture longer than bread made without them.

Mold, which sometimes forms on bread, is, like the yeast, a minute plant. It is floating about everywhere in the air, ready to settle down wherever it finds a suitable home. Moisture and heat favor its growth; hence bread should be thoroughly cooled before it is put into a jar or bread box. The bread box should be ventilated and kept in a cool place.

Rye bread contains a little more starch and less protein than wheat bread. It contains more water and holds its moisture longer.

Biscuits. The objection to eating hot bread does not hold for baking powder or soda biscuits, if well cooked, because these cool more rapidly and they do not contain the yeast plant; hence, they do not ferment as does the bread.

Baking powder is made from bicarbonate of soda (baking soda) and cream of tartar. When these are brought in contact with moisture, carbon dioxid is liberated, and in the effort to escape it causes the dough to expand and become light.

Breads made with pure baking powder are wholesome and, when light, are digestible. When made with cheap baking powder, however, in which alum or ammonia is employed, the stomach may be irritated by the chemical substances contained.

The reason that the cook attempts to bake her biscuits, or anything made with baking powder, as quickly as possible after the baking powder comes in contact with the moisture, is that the dough may have the full effect of the expansion of the gas. If the room in which she mixes her dough is cool, or if her biscuit dough is left in a cool place, this is not important, as heat and moisture are both required for full combustion. Enough baking powder biscuit dough may be mixed at one time to provide biscuits every morning for a week, if buried in flour immediately after mixing so that it is kept cool and from the air. A portion may be cut off each morning and the remainder again buried in the flour.

Macaroni and *spaghetti* are made from a special wheat flour known as Durum. They contain about seventy-seven per cent. of starch, little fat, and little protein. They may take the place of bread, rice, or potato at a meal.

Rice is a staple cereal in all tropical and temperate climates. It requires special machinery to remove the husk and the dark, outer skin of the kernel.

The polished rice commonly used, is almost pure starch, and, like white flour, lacks the nutritive qualities contained in the husk or covering.

It is seldom eaten within three months after harvesting and it is considered even better after two or three years. It requires thorough cooking.

Wild rice is used by the North American Indians. The seeds are longer, thinner, and darker, than the cultivated rice. It is coming into favor as a side dish but it is served more particularly at hotels in soup and with game.

As previously stated, rice contains a larger proportion of starch than any other cereal and the smallest proportion of protein. Next to rice, in starches, comes wheat flour; yet whole wheat or graham flour contain half as much again of protein.

Because of the quantity of starch in flour, potatoes, and rice, it is obvious that one should not eat freely of more than one of these at the same meal, else the digestive organs will be overworked in converting the starch into sugar, the liver overworked in converting the sugar into glycogen and back again into sugar, and be overloaded in storing it up.

By far the best plan is to eat but one cereal at a meal.

Rice contains no gluten, hence it cannot be raised in bread.

Unhusked rice is called paddy. The "vitamins" of rice are in the covering.

A German investigator, working to discover the cause of the disorder of nutrition known as "beri-beri" occurring in those who used polished rice freely, found that in those who used *un*polished rice, from which the outer husk had not been removed, the disease did not appear. He gave the name of "vitamin" to the substance in the outer husk, which prevented the disease.

While these substances were discovered while working with rice, they have since come to include other substances which affect the nutritive value of food. The term "vitamin" has since been given to other apparently necessary elements in foods which seem to determine their nutritive value to the system. These necessary elements, "vitamins," may be the spices and flavors used in the food, and sometimes, perhaps, may be the flavors resulting from the action of benign bacteria, as those which give the delicious flavor to butter and cheese.

Food, however nutritious, is lessened in its value to the system unless it appeals to the senses by its mode of preparation, seasoning, serving, and freshness. Sternberg insists that the senses of smell and taste determine chemical changes in foods with greater sensitiveness than chemical tests.

Dishes unskillfully prepared are not relished. Some chemical change has occurred which the senses detect and these dishes are rendered less wholesome, lacking the necessary "vitamin." Distaste, loss of appetite, and even nausea and vomiting may occur.

Sternberg calls attention anew to the fact that the science of cooking is a complicated one and is a matter of taste in the widest sense of the term, that vitamins may largely be produced in the preparation of the food.

Corn (maize) is a native of America and has been one of the most extensively used cereals.

The chief products of corn are hominy, corn meal, cracked corn, samp, glucose, corn-starch and laundry starch. Alcohol is also made from it.

Corn bread and corn-meal mush were important foods with the early settlers, partly because they are nutritious and partly because the corn meal was easily prepared at the mill and was cheap.

The germ of the corn is larger in proportion than the germs of other grains, and it contains much fat; therefore it is heating. For this reason, it is strange that corn bread is so largely used by inhabitants of the southern states. It is a more appropriate food for winter in cold climates.

Because of the fat in the germ, corn meal readily

turns rancid, and, on this account, the germ is separated and omitted from many corn-meal preparations.

Hulled corn, sometimes called lye hominy, is one of the old-fashioned ways of using corn. In its preparation, the skin is loosened by steeping the corn in a weak solution of lye, which gives it a peculiar flavor, pleasing to many.

Corn-meal mush is a valuable breakfast food if eaten with milk. If fried it should be covered with flour or dry corn meal and fried in deep fat, so that it does not soak up the fat.

Pop-corn. The bursting of the shell in popping corn is due to the expansion of the moisture in the starch, occasioned by the heat.

Green sweet corn does not contain the same proportion of starch as corn meal, it being, in its tender state, mostly water. It is laxative, because it is eaten with the coarse hull, which causes more rapid peristalsis of the intestines. It should be well masticated to break the covering of the husk; the digestive juices cannot penetrate the hard covering.

Breakfast Foods
The claims made for various advertised breakfast foods would be amusing if they were not intended to mislead. Nearly all of them have sufficient merit to sell them if the advertiser confines himself strictly to the truth, but the ever pertinent desire to excel, which is one great incentive to progress, leads to exaggeration. For example: the claim is sometimes made that they contain more nutriment than the same quantity of beef. Reference to Table V does not bear out such a statement. They contain more starch but less protein.

It is also claimed by some advertisers that breakfast foods are brain and nerve foods. The idea that certain foods are brain and nerve foods is erroneous, except that any tissue-building food (protein) builds nerve and brain tissue as it builds any other tissue, and the foods which produce heat and energy for other tissues produce the same for brain and nerve.

The grains commonly used for breakfast foods are corn, oats, rice, and wheat. Barley, and wild rice, millet and buckwheat are used in some sections, but not enough to warrant discussion here.

Barley is used chiefly for making malt and in the form of pearled barley is used in soups.

Table VI, from one of the bulletins published by the United States Department of Agriculture, is interesting from an economical standpoint.

TABLE VI

COMPARATIVE COST OF DIGESTIBLE NUTRIENTS AND AVAILABLE
ENERGY IN DIFFERENT CEREAL BREAKFAST FOODS

FOOD MATERIALS	Price per pound	Cost of one pound of protein	Cost of 1000 calories of energy	Amount for 10 cents				
				Total weight of material	Protein	Fat	Carbo-hydrates	Energy
Oat preparations:								
Oatmeal, raw	3	0.24	1.7	3.33	0.42	0.22	2.18	5884
"	4	0.32	2.3	2.50	0.31	0.16	1.64	4418
Rolled oats, steam cooked	6	0.48	3.4	1.67	0.21	0.11	1.08	2938
Wheat preparations:								
Flour, Graham	4	0.40	2.6	2.50	0.25	0.01	1.61	3790
Flour, entire-wheat	5	0.46	3.1	2.00	0.22	0.03	1.36	3188
Flour, patent	3.5	0.35	2.1	2.86	0.29	0.03	2.10	4700
Farina	10	1.12	6.2	1.00	0.09	0.01	0.73	1609

FOOD MATERIALS	Price per pound	Cost of one pound of protein	Cost of 1000 calories of energy	Amount for 10 cents				
				Total weight of material	Protein	Fat	Carbohydrates	Energy
Wheat Preparations—(*Continued*)								
Flaked	15	1.69	9.3	0.67	0.06	0.01	0.46	1005
Shredded	12.5	1.62	8.2	0.80	0.06	0.01	0.57	1217
Parched & ground	7.5	0.88	4.9	1.33	0.11	0.02	0.94	2050
Malted,cooked and crushed	13	1.43	8.5	0.77	0.07	0.01	0.53	1175
Flaked and malted	11	1.21	7.2	0.91	0.08	0.01	0.62	1389
Barley preparations:								
Pearled barley	7	1.06	4.6	1.43	0.09	0.01	1.04	2165
Flaked, steam cooked	15	1.83	9.6	0.67	0.05	...	0.50	1051
Corn preparations:								
Corn meal, granular	3	0.44	1.8	3.33	0.23	0.06	2.48	5534
Hominy	4	0.62	2.4	2.50	0.16	0.01	1.97	4178
Samp	5	0.78	3.0	2.00	0.13	0.01	1.57	3342
Flaked & parched	13	1.73	7.5	0.77	0.06	0.01	0.60	1335
Rice preparations:								
Rice, polished	8	1.48	4.7	1.25	0.07	...	0.94	1855
Flaked, steam cooked	15	2.31	9.8	0.67	0.04	...	0.51	1026
Miscellaneous foods for comparison:								
Bread, white	6	0.74	5.0	1.67	0.14	0.02	0.87	2009
"	5	0.62	4.2	2.00	0.16	0.02	1.04	2406
Crackers	10	1.10	5.3	1.00	0.09	0.08	0.71	1905
Macaroni	12.5	1.08	7.5	0.80	0.09	0.01	0.58	1328
Beans, dried	5	0.28	3.5	2.00	0.35	0.03	1.16	2868
Peas, dried	5	0.26	3.4	2.00	0.38	0.02	1.20	2974
Milk	3	0.94	9.7	3.33	0.11	0.13	0.17	1030
"	3.5	1.09	11.3	2.86	0.09	0.11	0.14	885
Sugar	5	...	2.8	2.00	...	...	2.00	3515
"	6	...	3.4	1.67	...	...	1.67	2940

The less expensive breakfast foods, such as oatmeal and corn meal, are as economical as flour, and, as they supply heat and energy in abundance, as shown by

Table VI, they should be supplied in the diet in proportion to the energy required. They are easily prepared for porridge, requiring simply to be boiled in water, with a little salt.

For invalids, children, and old people, breakfast foods prepared in gruels and porridges are valuable as they are easily digested. All should be thoroughly cooked so as to break the cell-walls inclosing the starch granules.

Oatmeal is the most nutritious cereal. The oat contains more fat than other grains and a larger proportion of protein. It, therefore, contains the proportion of nutrient elements best adapted to sustain life.

On account of the fat, oats are especially well adapted for a breakfast food in winter. Another advantage oatmeal, or rolled oats, have as a breakfast food is in their laxative tendency, due to the coarse shell of the kernel.

Oat breakfast foods keep longer than the foods made from wheat and rice.

There are no malts, or any mixtures in the oat preparations.

The difference between the various oatmeal breakfast foods is in their manner of preparation. They all contain the entire grain, with the exception of the husk. They are simply the ground or crushed oat. In preparing the oats before grinding, the outer hull is removed, the fuzzy coating of the berry itself is scoured off, the ends of the berry, particularly the end containing the germ, which is usually the place of deposit for insect eggs, is scoured, and the bitter tip end of the oat berry is likewise removed.

Rolled oats consist of the whole berry of the oat, ground into a coarse meal, either between millstones, or, in the case of the so-called "steel cut" oatmeal, cut with sharp steel knives across the sections of the whole oat groat.

Quaker Oats consist of the whole groats, which, after steaming in order to soften, have been passed between hot steel rolls, somewhat like a mangle in a laundry, and crushed into large, thin, partially cooked flakes. The oats are then further cooked by an open pan-drying process. This roasting process insures that all germ life is exterminated, renders the product capable of quicker preparation for the table, and causes the oil cells to release their contents, thereby producing what is termed the "nut flavor," which is not present in the old-fashioned type of oat product.

Both Rolled Oats and Quaker Oats are now partially cooked in their preparation, but the starch cells must be thoroughly broken and they should be cooked at least forty-five minutes in a double boiler; or, a good way to prepare the porridge is to bring it to the boiling point at night, let it stand covered over night and then cook it from twenty to thirty minutes in the morning. Another method of cooking is to bring the porridge to the boiling point and then place it in a fireless cooker over night.

The great fault in the preparation of any breakfast food is in not cooking it sufficiently to break the starch cells.

Puffed Rice is made from a good quality of finished rice. The process is a peculiar one, the outer covering or bran, is removed and then the product is literally "shot from guns"; that is, a quantity of the rice is placed in metal retorts, revolved slowly in an oven, at high temperature, until the pressure of steam, as shown by a gauge on the gun, indicates that the steam, generated slowly by the moisture within the grain itself, has thoroughly softened the starch cells. The gun retort is pointed into a wire cage and the cap which closes one end is removed, permitting an inrush of cold air. This cold air, on striking the hot steam, causes expansion, which amounts practically to an explosion. The expansion of steam within each starch cell completely shatters the cell, causing the grain to expand to eight times its original size. It rushes out of the gun and into the cage with great force, after which it is screened to remove all scorched or imperfectly puffed grains.

This process dextrinizes a portion of the starch and also very materially increases the amount of soluble material as against the original proportion in the grain.

Puffed Wheat is manufactured from Durum, or macaroni wheat, of the very highest grade. This is a very hard, glutinous grain. It is pearled in order to thoroughly clean and take off the outer covering of bran. It then goes through a puffing process, identical with that of Puffed Rice. The chemical changes are very similar to those of puffed rice.

Both Puffed Rice and Puffed Wheat are more digestible than in the original grain state. They are valuable foods for invalids.

Stale Bread. A food which tastes much like a prepared breakfast food, but is cheaper, may be made by dipping stale bread into molasses and water, drying it in the oven for several hours, and then crushing it. It is then ready to serve with cream. This is a palatable way to use up stale bread.

Crackers and Milk or Bread and Milk. As noted by Table VI, crackers are similar to breakfast food in nutrient elements, and with milk make a good food for breakfast, or a good luncheon. Business men, and others who eat hurriedly and return immediately to work, will do well to substitute crackers and milk, or bread and milk, for the piece of pie which often constitutes a busy man's lunch.

Cracked Wheat. In America wheat is seldom used whole. In England the whole grain, with the bran left on, is slightly crushed and served as cracked wheat or wheat grits.

Wheat is also rolled, or flaked, or shredded. The majority of wheat breakfast foods contain a part of the middlings and many of them bran. Farina and gluten preparations do not contain these, however.

The preparations of the various breakfast foods are a secret of the manufacturers. The ready-to-eat brands are cooked, then they are either rolled or shredded, the shredding requiring special machinery to tear the steamed kernels; later they are dried, and, finally packed, sometimes in small biscuits. Many preparations are baked after being steamed, which turns them darker and makes them more crisp. Some preparations are steamed, then run through rollers, while still wet, and pressed into flakes or crackers.

Predigested Foods. It is claimed that some foods are "partly digested and thus valuable for those with weak stomachs," but breakfast foods are largely starch and the starch is not digested by the gastric juice. It is digested by saliva and the ferments in the small intestine. These change the starch into dextrin and maltose.

Experiments with "predigested" foods do not show a larger proportion of dextrin (digested starch), however, than would naturally be produced by the heating of the starch when these foods are cooked at home.

The natural cooking makes starch more or less soluble, or at least gelatinized. As a result of these experiments therefore, the "predigested" argument is not of much weight.

Predigested foods, except in cases in which the patient is so weak as to be under the direction of a physician, are not desirable. Nature requires every organ to do the work intended for it, in order to keep up its strength, just as she requires exercise for the arms or legs to keep them strong. If an organ is weak, the *cause* must be found and corrected—perhaps the stomach or intestines need more blood, which should be supplied through exercise; or perhaps the nerves need relaxation; or the stomach less food; or food at more regular intervals.

Another argument against predigested foods lies in the fact that the chewing of coarse food is necessary to keep the teeth strong. For this strengthening of the teeth, children should be given dry crackers or dry toast each day.

Dogs and wild animals which chew bones and hard substances do not have pyorrhea, but lap-dogs and animals in the zoos, fed on bread and meat without bones, suffer from this disease.

In the so-called "predigested" or "malted" preparations, malt is added while they are being cooked.

Malt is a ferment made from some grain, usually from barley, the grain being allowed to germinate until the ferment diastase is developed.

There is no doubt that a number of foods containing malt are valuable to assist in converting starch into dextrin or sugar, just as pepsin is an aid in the digestion of protein; but eaten indiscriminately, there can be no question that it is more important for the teeth, stomach, and intestines to perform their natural work and thus keep their strength through normal exercise.

While they are not "predigested," as claimed, these foods are, as a rule, wholesome and nutritious. They are cleanly, and made from good, sound grain, and they contain no harmful ingredients. Some contain "middlings," molasses, glucose, and similar materials, but these are in no way injurious and have value as foods.

The dry, crisp, ready-to-eat foods are especially advantageous because of the mastication they require. This insures plenty of saliva being mixed with them to aid in digestion. A dish of such dry breakfast food, well masticated, together with an egg, to furnish a larger proportion of protein, makes a wholesome breakfast.

Cereal Coffees
According to investigations made by the United States Agriculture Experiment Station, cereal coffees are made of parched grains. A few contain a little true coffee, but for the most part they are made of parched wheat, barley, etc., or of grain mixed with wheat middlings, pea hulls, or corn cobs. There is no objection to any of these mixtures providing they are clean. The cereal coffees, as seen by Table VII, contain no more nourishment than the true coffee, but they are probably more easily digested; only a very little of the soluble starch passes into the water unless the kernel is ground. Coffee and tea are not taken for their nutrition, but for their stimulating effect on the nerves; and, if stimulation is desired, the cereal coffees fall short.

TABLE VII

COMPOSITION OF CEREAL–COFFEE INFUSION AND OTHER
BEVERAGES

KIND OF BEVERAGE	Water	Protein	Fat	Carbo-hydrates	Fuel Value per pound
Commercial cereal coffee (0.5 ounce to 1 pint water)	98.2	0.2	. . .	1.4	30
Parched corn coffee (1.6 ounces to 1 pint water)	99.5	0.2	. . . .	0.5	13
Oatmeal water (1 ounce to 1 pint water)	99.7	0.3	. . . .	0.3	11
Coffee (1 ounce to 1 pint water)	98.9	0.2	. . . .	0.7	16
Tea(0.5 ounce to 1 pint water)	99.5	0.2	. . . .	0.6	15
Chocolate (0.5 ounce to 1 pint milk)	84.5	3.8	4.7	6.0	365
Cocoa (0.5 ounce to 1 pint water)	97.1	0.6	0.9	1.1	65
Skimmed milk	88.8	4.0	1.8	5.4	170

By reference to Table VII it will be seen that cocoa and skimmed milk contain much more nutrition than any of the coffees. The chief value of cereal coffees is that they furnish a *warm* drink with the meal. They should not be too hot.

Barley or wheat, mixed with a little molasses, parched in the oven, and then ground, makes a mixture similar to the cereal coffee.

The old-fashioned crust coffee is just as nutritious as any of the coffees and has the advantage of being cheaper.

Barley water and oat water, made by boiling the ground kernel thoroughly and then straining, are nourishing foods for invalids and children. They are

6

often used as drinks by athletes and manual laborers, as they have the advantage of both quenching thirst and supplying energy.

Gruels are made in the same way, only strained through a sieve. This process allows more of the starch to pass with the water.

Legumes The legumes are the seeds of peas, beans, lentils, and peanuts.

TABLE VIII

LEGUMES

FOOD MATERIALS	Water per cent.	Protein per cent.	Fat per cent.	Carbo-hydrates per cent.	Ash per cent.	Fuel Value per pound Calories
Dried Legumes:						
Navy beans	12.6	22.5	1.8	59.6	3.5	1605
Dried peas	9.5	24.6	1.0	62.0	2.9	1655
Lentils	8.4	25.7	1.0	59.2	5.7	1620
Lima beans	10.4	18.1	1.5	65.9	4.1	1625
Peanuts	9.2	25.8	38.6	24.4	2.0	2560
Peanut butter	2.1	29.3	46.5	17.1	5.0	2825
Fresh Legumes:						
Canned peas	85.3	3.6	0.2	9.8	1.1	255
Canned lima beans	79.5	4.0	0.3	14.6	1.6	360
Canned string beans	93.7	1.1	0.1	3.8	1.3	95
Canned baked beans	68.9	6.9	2.5	19.6	2.1	600
String beans	89.2	2.3	0.3	7.4	0.8	195
Shelled peas	74.6	7.0	0.5	16.9	1.0	465

Like the cereals, they are seeds, yet they contain a very much larger proportion of protein and may be substituted for meat or eggs in a diet. In all vegetarian diets, under normal conditions, the legumes should be used freely to replace meats.

All legumes must be thoroughly cooked and thoroughly masticated. Because the protein in these foods is less digestible than that in meat or eggs, particularly if they are not thoroughly masticated, they are better adapted for the use of those who do manual labor. Soldiers in battle, day laborers, and others whose work calls for hard physical exercise, can digest legumes more easily than can those whose occupation is more sedentary.

If not thoroughly masticated legumes usually produce intestinal fermentation with consequent production of gas. For this reason they occasion distress in those who partake of them too freely and with insufficient preparation by cooking.

The protein of the legumes is of the same nature as the casein of milk. It has been called vegetable casein.

Peanuts. While an underground vegetable, grown like potatoes, peanuts resemble nuts, inasmuch as they contain so much fat. The extracted oil is used in several commercial products.

Like other legumes, they require cooking. They are roasted because this develops the flavor.

Because they contain a more balanced proportion of proteins, carbohydrates, and fats, they will sustain life for some time without other food, as they provide rebuilding material, energy, and heat. Used alone, however, there is no counteracting acid, and it is better to add some fruit, such as apples, or apples and dates. For this reason lemon juice is mixed with peanut butter.

In eating peanuts it is imperative that they be masticated *until they are a pulp*, otherwise they are very difficult of digestion. The pain which many people experience after eating peanuts is probably due to eating too large a quantity and not fully masticating them, forgetting that they are a very rich, highly concentrated food.

The habit of eating peanuts between meals and then eating a hearty meal is likely to overload the digestive organs.

Both peanuts and peanut butter contain over twenty-five per cent. of protein and about thirty-nine per cent. of fat; therefore they yield much heat and energy.

Peanuts have been made into a flour; they are also to be had in the form of grits which are cooked like oatmeal.   When nuts or peanuts are used as an after-dinner relish the quantity of meat should be cut down.

Their popularity is evidenced by the fact that between 4,000,000 and 5,000,000 bushels are raised annually in America.

Peanut Butter.   While peanut butter contains 46.5 per cent. fat, it contains only seventeen per cent. carbohydrates.   Since sugars and starches are protections to fat, being used for energy before the fats are consumed, if these sugars and starches are not supplied in other food, the fats in the peanut butter are consumed for energy.   If starches *are* consumed in other foods, it is clear that one who wishes to reduce in flesh should avoid peanut butter, as well as other fats.

Peanut butter is more easily digested than the roasted peanut, unless the latter is chewed to a pulp. It can be made at home by grinding the peanuts in a meat grinder, and then further mashing with a rolling pin or a wooden potato masher.   A little lemon juice mixed with the peanut butter makes it not only more palatable, but more easily digested.   A peanut butter sandwich is quite as nourishing as a meat sandwich.

Shelled Peas. Shelled peas were used in Europe as far back as in the Middle Ages, and there, to-day, the dried or "split" pea is used quite as extensively as the dried bean. In America, peas are used almost entirely in the green stage, fresh, or canned.

As seen by Table VIII, the green, shelled pea contains seven per cent. of protein and sixteen per cent. of sugar and starch, while the dry or "split" pea contains over 24.5 per cent. of protein and sixty-two per cent. of sugar and starch, the difference being in the amount of water contained in the shelled peas. Canned peas contain even a larger percentage of water.

A variety of the pea is now being cultivated, in which, like the string bean, the pod is used as a food. They are sweet and delicious.

Dried peas are used in this country mostly in purées.

Beans. Baked navy beans may well be substituted on a menu for meat, containing, as they do, 22.5 per cent. of protein. It is needless to state that beans and lean meat or eggs should not be served at the same meal. Beans have the advantage of being cheaper than meat, yet, as stated above, the protein in the legumes is less easily digested than the protein of meat or eggs. They must be thoroughly cooked and thoroughly masticated.

There is but a small percentage of fat in dried beans; for this reason they are usually baked with a piece of pork. They make a very complete, perhaps the most complete food, containing nutrient elements in about the proper proportions.

A bean biscuit is used for the sustenance of soldiers on a march; it gives a complete food in condensed form.

In baking dried beans or peas, soft or distilled water should be used, as the lime of hard water makes the shell almost indigestible. Parboiling the beans for fifteen minutes in two quarts of water with a quarter of a teaspoon of baking soda softens the shell, making them easier to digest.

String Beans. The string bean contains very little nutrition, as shown by Table VIII. The pod and the bean, at this unripe stage, contain nearly ninety per cent. water. Their chief value as a food consists in their appetizing quality to those who are fond of them, thus stimulating the flow of gastric juice.

Like all green vegetables they stimulate the action of the kidneys. All green vegetables are particularly valuable to those who drink little water.

The dried *Lima* bean, used during the winter, may be boiled or baked. If old, they are practically indigestible.

Kidney Beans contain much water but are more nutritious than the string bean.

Soy Bean. In China and Japan this bean is used extensively. Being rich in protein, used with rice it makes a well-balanced diet.

The soy bean is made into various preparations, one of the most important being *shoyo*, which has been introduced into other countries. To make it, the soy bean is cooked and mixed with roasted wheat flour and salt; into this is put a special ferment. It is then allowed to stand for an extended time in casks. The result is a thick, brown liquid with a pungent, agreeable taste. It is very nourishing.

A kind of cheese is also made by boiling the soy bean for several hours, wrapping the hot mass in bundles of straw, and putting it in a tightly closed cellar for twenty-four hours.

Lentils are not commonly used in this country, but they were one of the earliest vegetables to be cultivated in Asia and the Mediterranean countries. They are usually imported and may be obtained in the markets. They are used like dried peas and are fully as nourishing, but the flavor of the lentil is pronounced and they are not so agreeable to the average person as peas or beans.

Nuts are classed with the carbo-nitrogenous foods, because of the more nearly **Nuts** equal proportion of proteins and carbonaceous substances.

TABLE IX

NUTS

FOOD MATERIALS	Water per cent.	Protein per cent.	Fat per cent.	Carbohydrates per cent.	Ash per cent.	Fuel Value per pound Calories.
Almonds	4.8	21.0	54.90	17.3	2.0	3030
Brazil nuts	5.3	17.0	66.80	7.0	3.9	3329
Filberts	3.7	15.6	65.30	13.0	2.4	3342
Hickory nuts	3.7	15.4	67.40	11.4	2.1	3495
Pecans	3.0	16.7	71.20	13.3	1.5	3633
English walnuts	2.8	16.7	64.40	14.8	1.3	3305
Chestnuts, fresh	45.0	6.2	5.40	42.1	1.3	1125
Walnuts, black	2.5	27.6	56.30	11.7	1.9	3105
Cocoanut, shredded	3.5	6.3	57.30	31.6	1.3	3125
Peanuts, roasted	1.6	30.5	49.20	16.2	2.5	3177

It will be noted, by reference to Table IX that nuts contain a much larger proportion of fats and less starch than the legumes.   Chestnuts contain the largest amount of starch, and pecans the most fat.

Peanuts are classed here with nuts because of their similar use in the diet.   Their comparative richness in protein will be noted.

Nuts are a valuable food, but they should be made a part of a meal and may well take the place of meat rather than eaten as a dessert, because of the large percentage of protein.   They are too rich to be eaten as a relish at the end of a meal, if one has eaten as much other food as the system requires.

In planning a meal, if the dietary is rich in starches and lacking in protein, a side dish of nuts may be served.

Too great stress cannot be laid on the importance of the thorough mastication of nuts; otherwise they are difficult of digestion.   When thoroughly chewed, however, they are as easily digested as cereals or legumes.   If ground fine in a meat grinder or rubbed through a sieve, they digest more readily, but this grinding does not take the place of the grinding with the teeth and the mixture with the saliva.   They are best chopped for salads, cake, or croquettes.   When ground the oil extracted makes them pasty and not appetizing in appearance for use in salads or cake.

Milk   Milk is a perfect food for the infant because it contains the elements in proper proportions to sustain life and growth, though, alone, it is insufficient for the nourishment of healthy adults. The adult, in order to get sufficient nutriment, would be compelled to take a larger proportion of water than necessary, the proportion of water required by the system being about sixty-seven per cent., while milk contains eighty-seven per cent.

In many diseases, however, a whole or partial milk diet is desirable, especially in any inflammatory condition of the gastro-intestinal tract.

TABLE X

MILK AND MILK PRODUCTS

FOOD MATERIALS	Water	Protein	Fats	Sugar	Salts	Lactic Acid
Milk	86.8	4.0	3.7	4.8	0.7	....
Skimmed milk	88.0	4.0	1.8	5.4	0.8	....
Buttermilk	90.6	3.8	1.2	3.3	0.6	0.3
Cream	66.0	2.7	26.7	2.8	1.8	....
Cheese	36.8	33.5	24.3	....	5.4	....
Butter	6.0	0.3	91.0	....	2.7	....

The milk of the cow is not perfectly adapted for the young child—it is lacking in the proper proportion of sugar, and when fed to the infant it must be modified. Mother's milk is not only richer in sugar than cow's milk, but it contains about half as much casein. The calf needs more albumin than the baby does because it grows faster. Human milk is also richer in fat.

An all-milk diet may be followed when it is desirable to gain in weight. Such a diet should be accompanied by exercises for the vital organs and by deep breathing, but experiments have shown that healthy digestive organs do their work better when a part of the food is solid.

A milk and cream diet of about three quarts milk and one quart cream with the addition of one to two eggs a day will keep up the strength of one in bed, but is not sufficient for one who is active.

In order for an adult to obtain the proper quantity of carbohydrates and fat, from an all-milk diet, it is necessary for him to drink from four to five quarts of milk a day (sixteen to twenty glasses). It is usually said that on an all-milk diet an active person requires as many quarts as he is feet tall.

Young babies on mother's milk are almost always fat, because of the larger proportion of sugar and fat in the mother's milk.

Reference to Table X shows that the thirteen per cent. of solids are about equally divided between fat, sugar, and protein. The sugar is lactose. It supplies heat to the infant before it can exercise its muscles vigorously. The protein is casein.

There is no starch in milk. The digestive ferment, which acts on starch, has not developed in the young babe and it cannot digest starch.

The salts promote the growth of bone.

The fat in milk is in small emulsified droplets within a thin albuminous sheath. When allowed to stand in a cool place it rises to the top.

Besides casein, milk contains a certain amount of albumin—about one-seventh of the total amount—called lactalbumin. It maintains the fat in milk in emulsified form.

In young babes the milk is curdled in the stomach, or the casein separated from the water and sugar, not by hydrochloric acid, but by a ferment in the gastric juice, known as rennin. Rennin, or rennet, from the stomachs of calves, is used in cheese and butter factories to coagulate the casein. This with other chemicals so hardens the casein that it is used in the manufacture of buttons.

Preserving milk. If milk could be kept free from bacteria, it would keep sweet almost indefinitely. At the Paris Exposition, milk from several American dairies was kept sweet for two weeks, without any preservative except cleanliness and a temperature of about forty degrees. The United States Bureau of Animal Industry states that milk may be kept sweet for seven weeks without the use of chemicals.

The importance of absolute cleanliness in the preparation and marketing of this important article of food is being recognized both by the producer and the consumer, and careful inspection has done away with many abuses. In the absence of an efficient health department, the consumer should ascertain in every case how the milk he uses is handled at every stage before it reaches him. Care in this regard may safeguard his family from disease and save him many dollars.

The best method for the housewife to follow is to keep the milk clean, cool, and away from other foods, as milk will absorb a bad odor or flavor from any stale food or odorous vegetables, from fresh paint, or other substances.

Milk must never be left exposed in a sick room or in a refrigerator unless the waste pipe and the ice chamber are kept scrupulously clean.

Milk Tests. In testing the value of milk, or the value of a cow, butter makers and farmers gauge it by the amount of butter fat in the milk, while the cheese maker tests the milk for the proportion of protein (casein). The amount of butter fat depends on the feed and water, and on the breed. If the total nutrient elements fall below twelve per cent., it is safe to assume that the milk has been watered.

In cheese and butter there is no sugar; it remains in the buttermilk and the whey, both of which the farmer takes home from the factories to fatten his hogs.

Pasteurized Milk. In pasteurizing milk the aim is to destroy as many of the bacteria as possible without causing any chemical changes or without changing the flavor. One can pasteurize milk at home by placing it in an air-tight bottle, immersing the bottle to the neck in hot water, heating the water to 167 F. for twenty minutes, and then quickly cooling the milk to 50 F. by immersing the bottle in cold water. The rapid cooling lessens the cooked taste. The best dairies pasteurize the milk before it is marketed.

Sterilized Milk. Milk is sterilized to destroy all bacteria, by heating it to 212 F. Sterilized milk remains sweet longer than pasteurized milk, but more chemical changes are produced and the flavor is changed, resembling that of boiled milk.

Formerly borax, boric acid, salicylic acid, formalin, and saltpeter were used to keep the milk sweet, but this adulteration is now forbidden by the pure-food laws.

Malted milk is a dry, soluble food product in powder form, derived from malted barley, wheat flour (dextrin), and cow's milk, containing the full amount of cream.

The process of the extraction from the cereals is conducted at elevated temperatures so as to allow the active agents (enzymes) of the barley malt to effect the conversion of the vegetable protein and starches. The filtered extract, containing the derivatives of the malt, wheat, and the full-cream cow's milk, is then evaporated to dryness *in vacuo*, the temperature being controlled so as to obviate any alteration of the natural constituents of the ingredients and so as to preserve their full physiological values. The strictest precautions are observed to insure the purity of the product. It contains:

```
Fats................................................   8.75
Proteins...........................................  16.35
Dextrin............................................  18.80
Lactose and Maltose...............................  49.15
    (Total Soluble Carbohydrates)..................  67.95
Inorganic Salts....................................   3.86
Moisture...........................................   3.06
```

Malted milk is free from germs. The starches and sugars are converted in the process of manufacture into maltose, dextrin, and lactose. The fats are in an absorbable condition, and it contains a high percentage of proteins derived from both the milk and the grains, as well as a marked percentage of mineral salts. It is readily soluble in water and is easily digested.

The hydrochloric acid of the stomach coagulates or curds milk much as it is curded by many fruit and vegetable acids, such as those in lemons or tomatoes. Thus the milk forms into curds immediately on entering the stomach, the casein being at once precipitated by the rennin. This is the chief reason why it should be drunk slowly, otherwise too large curds will form, causing distress from pressure.

A part of the digestion of the casein is performed by pepsin in the stomach and a part by the trypsin of the pancreatic juice.   Digestion of Milk

The larger part of the digestion of the milk sugar or lactose, is performed by the pancreatic juice; although it is partly acted on by the saliva. Usually, however, the saliva is given little chance to become mixed with the milk, unless it is taken slowly and mixed with saliva by chewing movements. This is one reason why children should be given milk in which bread has been broken, rather than a piece of bread and a glass of milk. By swallowing the milk slowly, smaller curds are formed in the stomach and the milk is more thoroughly digested.

The salts of milk, to a large extent, the water, and perhaps a portion of the sugar are absorbed in the stomach.

When the fat (cream) is removed milk digests more readily, so that in cases in which the stomach is delicate, *skimmed milk, clabbered milk, or buttermilk* are often prescribed instead of sweet milk.

Boiled milk is also more readily digested by some; the lactalbumin is separated and rises to the top in a crinkly scum. The casein of boiled milk is also more readily digested, forming in small flakes in the stomach instead of in curds.

Sterilizing the milk by boiling will prevent the action of bacteria in producing fermentation and disordered digestion, and, if relished, milk can thus be treated. Pasteurized milk is more palatable than boiled milk.

Milk is often better assimilated if other food is not too suddenly cut off. When the diet is radically changed the digestive system is apt to show derangement. Therefore when for any cause an all-milk diet is desired, it is unwise to begin it at once, by feeding from eighteen to twenty glasses of milk a day. This amount may be approximated within a week's time. The change in diet should be begun by cutting down all meats and legumes and gradually eliminating

starches. In changing from a milk diet to a diet
including more hearty foods, the transition should
also be gradual.

If a milk diet is to be followed and the milk seems
to disturb the stomach when taken in quantities, one
may begin by taking it in very small quantities every
fifteen minutes for the first hour. If one's purpose is
to gain in flesh the quantity may be increased to a
glass, and time intervals be lengthened to every hour
as the stomach becomes accustomed to caring for the
milk. It should be sipped slowly and thoroughly
mixed with saliva before being swallowed. The
mouth should be carefully rinsed with equal parts of
peroxide of hydrogen and water, or listerine and hot
sterile water, each time milk is taken.

Milk, in whatever form it is taken, leaves a coating
on the tongue and teeth. The heat of the mouth,
especially if the patient is feverish, quickly causes
changes which give a disagreeable taste and a chance
for bacterial action. These bacterial products are
carried into the stomach and excite digestive changes
through which fermentation and gas formation appear
and biliousness may result. This may be avoided if,
after taking the milk, the mouth is carefully washed
and, in feverish conditions, the tongue gently scraped
or swabbed with absorbent cotton dipped in listerine
or peroxide of hydrogen. Without such cleansing of
the mouth milk may disagree.

When from two to three glasses of milk at a meal are
taken, less solid food is needed, because the required
nutriment is partially supplied by the milk. One
reason why milk seems to disagree with many people,
is because they lose sight of the fact that milk is an
actual food, as well as a beverage, and they eat the

usual quantity of food in addition to the milk.   As
one pint, or two glasses of milk, contains approximately
the same amount of nutrition as one-third of a pound
of beef, the amount of food to be taken in addition
may be readily calculated.

The chief reason for the lessened activity of the
bowels on a milk diet is because the nourishment in
milk is practically all absorbed—there is very little
residue and milk gives little rough surface to excite
peristaltic action and stimulate the walls of the
intestine to activity.

The calcium, one of the constituents of milk, tends
to lessen the peristaltic action of the intestines and
this is one of the causes of constipation.   Fruit and
coarse bread containing much bran, should be used
with a milk diet.

Constipation may also be occasioned by drinking
milk rapidly.   When the hydrochloric acid is very
active coagulation may take place so quickly as to
cause hard tough curds to form; these enter the intestine undissolved because the gastric juice can act
only on the exterior portion; the stomach retains the
curds in its effort to dissolve them and fermentation
may occur, with irritation and constipation from irregular action.   In this case the constipating effect
may be overcome by taking the milk in small sips or
by the addition of one part of lime-water to six parts
milk.   The lime-water causes the curds to be precipitated in small flakes.

Lime-water may be prepared by putting a heaping
teaspoon of unslaked lime with a quart of boiled or
distilled water into a corked bottle or Mason jar.
Shake thoroughly two or three times during the first
hour; then allow the lime to settle, and after twenty-

four hours pour or siphon off the clear fluid. Be careful not to allow the lime to be poured off with the water.

Barley water or oatmeal water added to milk also prevents the formation of large curds.

Milk may also be taken with any variety of gruel —oatmeal, sago, arrowroot, or tapioca.

If there is much mucus in the stomach, mucous fermentation may occur in milk because of the lack of hydrochloric acid. The partially digested curds are tough, stringy, and slimy and the intestinal walls find no resistance in the mass. In this case constipation may be followed by diarrhea.

If the stomach is deficient in hydrochloric acid the juice of half an orange or a little lemon juice may be taken a half hour before the glass of milk.

Constipation and, later, diarrhea may also result when stomach digestion is weak, the curds passing through the stomach and intestines undissolved.

When there is any tendency to torpidity of the liver, daily exercise should be directed to the liver, stomach, and intestines or milk may cause biliousness, because the excess of fat and protein taken over-stimulates the liver, causing an excess of bile. The bile may enter the stomach and cause nausea and vomiting. Constipation results from the disordered digestion. This will not often occur if one exercises daily and cuts down the quantity of solid food as the amount of liquid is increased.

A glass of hot Vichy or Hunyadi water taken the first thing on rising, and followed by a glass of cool water will help to relieve any engorgement of the liver.

In case of biliousness resulting from a milk diet,

abstain from all food for twenty-four hours, cleanse the mouth as indicated above, and drink freely of water.

When the liver is a little inactive, milk may be diluted with an aerated water or even plain water. Daily exercise directed toward securing a greater activity of the liver and gall-bladder should be followed. Four tablespoonfuls of soda water, Apollinaris, or carbonic-acid water to the glass may be used.

As noted in the preceding pages, orange and lemon juice will encourage greater activity of the stomach and bowels.

One-third of a glass of hot Vichy water to each glass of milk renders it easily digested and most people relish it. Unless the liver is very inactive milk taken in this way will not constipate and exercise directed to the liver, as previously mentioned, will help to obviate this condition.

Skimmed milk, Kumyss, or buttermilk are easily digested and are valuable when the digestive system is weak.

The monotony of a milk diet tends to create a distaste for milk and the mental revolt may upset digestion and result in constipation. This should be kept in mind and various ways of modifying the milk be used to create variety; mental aversion and antagonism should be corrected.

When its taste is not relished milk may be made acceptable and the stomach induced to retain it by using a variety of flavors. A drop or two of vanilla, a trifle of cinnamon, nutmeg, salt and pepper, chocolate, or any other flavor that is liked may be used, varying them so as to keep from monotony.

If milk seems to produce gas in the stomach with

distress and the milk is retained too long in the stomach from the interference with its movements caused by the gas, a teaspoonful of malt extract may be added to each glass of milk. If the malt extract is not at hand, four teaspoonfuls of malted milk to each glass may be used.

Equal parts of cream and hot water to which has been added a third of a teaspoon of soda may be used, for the same purpose.

If milk disagrees because of an excess of hydrochloric acid and the formation of hard curds, a saltspoon of salt or bicarbonate of soda may be used, or one part of lime-water to six parts of milk.

When milk seems to disagree because digestion is somewhat slow and the milk does not offer enough bulk to excite peristaltic action, it remains too long in the stomach and fermentation occurs. A slice of bread, a couple of crackers, a piece of zweiback, a tablespoonful of Nestle's or Mellin's food or of arrow-root gruel added to each glass, or eaten with the milk, will give it more body and prevent the formation of large curds.

When the stomach is excessively weak because of a lack of the digestive juices and a consequent incomplete action of the stomach, only predigested milk should be taken until the stomach has been brought to a normal tone. Pepsin or pancreatin may be used for the partial digestion. Milk so predigested must be freshly prepared each time it is used or must be kept on ice until used. The stomach will find practically no difficulty in assimilating milk thus prepared, and constipation will be avoided.

It must be remembered that milk must be sipped slowly and be well mixed with saliva before it is swallowed.

Milk can be soured and taken separated as a variation, the curds and whey being relished by many when properly prepared. A little sugar and cinnamon or nutmeg sprinkled on curds or mixed with the whey make a palatable mixture. Buttermilk or kumyss offer still other variations.

With all these means of varying the taste, appearance, or condition of milk it is hardly possible that some way cannot be found whereby milk may be taken and be well borne by the stomach and the full benefits from its use be derived.

Cheese   This is the casein (protein) which has been separated from milk by the action of rennet. It is highly nutritious and many varieties are on the market. In Europe it is largely used to take the place of meat. Cheese contains almost as much again protein as is contained in the same quantity of meat.

In this country more highly flavored cheeses are in demand, and when eaten in moderate quantities they aid digestion. They are highly concentrated food and but a small quantity should be eaten at a meal, particularly if meat has constituted a part of the meal.

The cheeses poor in fat are more difficult to digest as they are harder and not so easily masticated.

Contrary to the prevalent idea, a properly made Welsh rarebit is more easily digested than uncooked cheese.

One should use judgment, in eating any highly concentrated food, not to eat too large a quantity.

Smierkase, or cottage cheese, is coagulated casein. It contains thirty-three per cent. of protein, twenty-four per cent. of fat, and five per cent. of salts.

The thickening of the milk, or the coagulation of the casein, is like that produced by lactic acid.

Skimmed milk, as shown by the table, contains the same amount of protein as fresh milk, but more sugar and more ash, the difference consisting almost entirely of less fat, which has been removed in the cream.

Buttermilk. There is less fat, protein, sugar, or ash in buttermilk than in skimmed milk; it is therefore less nourishing, but it requires less digestive effort. The sugar has partially fermented and the lactic acid is freed. It is the free lactic acid which gives the pungent taste.

Buttermilk made by lactone or Bulgarian tablets and fresh milk is as nourishing and as desirable as that made in the process of butter making, and it has the advantage of being fresh. When the whole milk is used it, of course, contains the same amount of fat, protein, sugar, and ash as the milk. It is of value in cases of poor digestion of protein and fat, and in chronic stomach trouble. It has been claimed that the bacilli in buttermilk made from the Bulgarian tablets prevent putrefaction in the large intestine. This is disputed, however.

Clabbered Milk. The casein in clabbered milk coagulates and if kept in a hot place the coagulation continues until the water, sugar, and salts are separated. Clabbered or loppered milk is wholesome. It may be sweetened or salted and flavored to taste.

Whey is the watery portion of milk from which the casein has been removed in the process of making cheese. It is a palatable drink and may be flavored with a little nutmeg and sugar or salt. Invalids

usually relish it.   Beef tea or egg yolk may be added
to it.

Milk Sugar.   Sugar made from milk is now a commercial product; it is evaporated and transformed
into a fine powder.   This powder is used by physicians and druggists in compounding powders, pills,
tablets, etc.

Junket.   The tablets used in making junket are
the essence of rennet.   Milk coagulated by rennin
has not the sour taste of milk coagulated by acid.
It is an admirable article of diet in many weakened
conditions of the digestive tract.

Condensed Milk is made by evaporating the water
until it is reduced to about sixty-one per cent.   It is
then hermetically sealed.   It is convenient for use
whenever fresh milk cannot be obtained, but the
process of evaporation changes its flavor so that few
care for it as a drink.   It may be substituted for
cream in coffee, and diluted with three times its volume
in water the proportions are again the same as before
the water was evaporated.

CHAPTER IV

B EVERAGES are used primarily to relieve thirst;
they may also contain food elements; they may
be used for their effect in heat and cold, for their
flavor, which helps to increase the appetite, or for
their stimulating properties.

They are used to aid digestion and the elimination
of waste, to promote sweating, to soothe inflamed
air passages or digestive membranes. They furnish
extra nutrition, stimulate nerve action, quench thirst
in fevers, warm the body when it is cold or cool it
when it is hot. They are used in health or disease,
from the snows of the arctics to the palms of the tropics.
They may be alkaline or acid, mineral, medicated or
mucilaginous, effervescing or plain. The question of
their utility and preparation is important in any
discussion of foods and food products, though in
themselves they are not foods.

The people of all races seemingly crave a stimulant,
after bodily or mental exertion, in fatigue, as a
"bracer" in prolonged effort, as a promoter of
sociability, or as an offering of hospitality. These
stimulants are either alcoholic or non-alcoholic.

It is a notable fact that no tribe is so remote that
it does not possess some form of beverage which may

be offered to friends or used to promote feelings of conviviality; or it may be used to stir up rage if onslaughts against neighboring tribes are contemplated. The craving is universal and as old as the race.

Those who decry this craving when it takes the form of alcohol are often themselves addicted to excessive drinking of non-alcoholic stimulants.

Tea   Tea is not a food—it is a stimulant. It is made by steeping the leaves of a shrub, called Thea, which grows in the tropical regions of Asia and adjacent islands.

Green tea differs from black in the mode of its preparation. In green tea the leaves are steamed before they are dried.

The amount of tannin in green tea is greater than in black, hence green tea is regarded as not so wholesome a drink as black tea.

The young tender leaves are more delicate of flavor.

Varieties of plants differ both in the amount of tannin and the delicacy of flavor.

Tea should never be boiled or allowed to stand longer than a few minutes; standing causes the tannin to be extracted from the leaves, and this tannin disturbs digestion. It is the tannin extracted from the bark of trees which toughens animal skins into leather.

The best way to make tea is to pour on boiling water and serve within five minutes.

Because of the uncertainty as to the length of time tea may be allowed to steep in hotel kitchens or restaurants, it is a wise custom to have a ball of tea and a pot of hot water served that the guest may make the tea at the table.

Tea is diuretic, stimulating the action of the kidneys. Through its stimulant action it relieves fatigue and has been found especially useful in Arctic explorations and for soldiers on long marches.

When taken hot it will often relieve sick headache. When taken on an empty stomach, after a long fatiguing tramp or a prolonged "shopping" excursion, its refreshing effect may be felt for an hour or two.

The ease of its preparation and the quickness of its effect tends to produce the "tea habit." When drunk to excess with meals, it causes the precipitation of the ferments in the digestive juices, retards digestion, and may cause constipation, particularly if taken after long infusion.

Strong tea has an overstimulating effect on the nervous system which reacts, producing depression and restlessness; this may lead to insomnia, muscular twitchings, and palpitation of the heart.

Habitual users often take from ten to twenty cups of strong tea daily; in these the evil effects of the tea habit are easily noted.

Americans, or any people whose nerves are highly stimulated, from the stress of life, or from habitual nerve tension, should particularly avoid all stimulating beverages.

Poor tea, because of the greater amount of tannin it contains, produces its ill effects more quickly. From overstimulation of the nervous system, poor tea, long stewed, has been held to be a contributing factor in insanity.

Tea should be avoided by the dyspeptic, by those of constipated and flatulent habit, or by the anemic.

Tannin coagulates the albumin in milk or cream and the addition of these to tea renders it more indigestible; plain or with lemon juice it may be well borne by those with whom it disagrees when used with cream or sugar.

Thein, the active principle in tea, is chemically identical with caffein in coffee.

Coffee Coffee is prepared from the seeds of the coffee tree. The best known brands come from the Island of Java, Mocha, Rio de Janeiro, and Mexico.

Coffee, like tea, *is not a food*, it is a stimulant.

The active principle is caffein. This is an alkaloid and is a strong stimulant to the central nervous system. It quickens the heart action, and the stimulating effect is so apparent with many, that they cannot sleep for several hours after drinking it. Others drink coffee to quicken mental activity and to keep them awake.

It must be borne in mind, however, that there is a reactionary effect from all stimulants, and while coffee is not intoxicating, as alcohol, it has a similar effect on the nerves and heart.

Coffee has the redeeming feature of having a pleasing aroma, which, because of the effect on the mind, may incite the flow of gastric juice. Despite the fact that no morning beverage has quite the same pleasing aroma, or pungency, ordinarily one is much better without it.

Coffee stimulates the action of the heart and for this reason it is used in collapse to restore heart action.

It removes the sense of fatigue and is thus beneficial in some cases, as in the army, when long marches are necessary.

It is valuable as an antidote in opium poisoning or in cases of alcoholism.

It is given to those addicted to liquor, as a milder stimulant when they are recovering from a spell of intoxication.

The only use of coffee as a food is that its pleasant aroma stimulates the flow of gastric juice.

Strong coffee, particularly that which has been boiled for a long time, retards digestion, and, if much is drunk, it will produce the same symptoms of over stimulation of the nervous system as are manifest in the tea habit. Heartburn, constipation, dyspepsia, and insomnia may result.

Sometimes the habit is manifested by excessive eating of the coffee bean. Such users show marked symptoms of nervousness; they are usually thin and their faces are drawn and anxious.

Each person must decide for himself whether or not coffee or tea is injurious to him and cease the habit if he finds it is interfering with the proper functioning of the system, remembering always that the purpose of food is to resupply body waste and produce heat and energy.

One who knows that coffee disturbs his digestion, and yet cannot break himself from the habit of drinking it, should have sympathy for the one who is addicted to liquor and finds it difficult to break the habit of depending on this *so-called* stimulant.

Cereal Coffee has been discussed under the heading "Cereals."

"Crust" coffee is made by pouring boiling water on "caramelized" bread or bread deeply toasted, allowing it to stand ten minutes, then pouring off the liquid, which may be sweetened to taste or mixed with cream or milk. It is also made by using crusts of bread which have been dried in the oven without being allowed to brown.

Cocoa and Chocolate *Cocoa and Chocolate* are prepared from the cocoa bean.

Cocoa is from the shell of the bean and chocolate from the kernel. As shown by Table VII, they are more nutritious than the other beverages.

Cocoa butter is the fat of the cocoa bean. It has a pleasant odor and does not easily become rancid. Its nutritive value depends on its fat.

Most of the fat has been removed from the cocoa made for the use of invalids, hence the nutritive value of this cocoa is lessened. The milk and sugar used in its preparation constitute the most of its nourishment; the cocoa simply gives a flavor.

Part of the value of chocolate is in the sugar used with it. If well prepared it is digested with ease and forms a nutritious article of diet. The habit of using large amounts of chocolate in candy, or as a beverage, disorders the system because of the gastric disturbances produced by the excess of sugar.

When food is not easily obtained, compressed cakes of chocolate may be carried, as in traveling, for a temporary food supply.

Chocolate, as sugar, in moderation, constitutes a good food for the growing child.

The active principle in cocoa and chocolate is *theobromin* and, though milder, is similar to caffein in its stimulating effect on the nervous system.

Lemonade *Lemonade* and other fruit drinks, particularly those made from the citrus fruits, slake the thirst more quickly than most drinks.

All fruit drinks are diuretic, and, whenever the action of the kidneys is sluggish, they are especially desirable.

These are made by forcing carbon dioxid, under pressure, into the bottle. As soon as the cork is removed the escape of the gas causes effervescence. These drinks are of no special advantage, other than that they slake the thirst, because the amount of salts of various minerals they contain is usually small.

Effervescing Waters

When taken in excess they cause flatulence and may lead to gastric disturbances. The indiscriminate habit of young people drinking effervescing waters at soda fountains should be discouraged.

These waters added to milk render it more easily digested.

There is no beverage nor concoction devised by man equal to water. It is to be deplored that it is not used as freely as Nature demands—from eight to ten glasses a day.

Water

The value of water as a food and as an aid to digestion is discussed on page 26.

CONDIMENTS

Condiments are not foods. They have no nutrition in themselves, but by their flavor they stimulate the nerves of taste, rendering the food more appetizing and help to make the diet more varied.

They are relishes and are to be employed in this manner judiciously, and not used generally in the diet.

Some strong condiments, as cayenne pepper, are of use in dyspeptic conditions to stimulate the gastric mucous membrane.

They are of value in the dietary of the invalid whose appetite must be stimulated and careful variations in flavoring will aid in varying a diet which otherwise would be monotonous, but the excessive use of condiments, particularly the various peppers, salt, horseradish, ginger, vinegar, and spices, as indulged by many, so overstimulates the gastric and intestinal membranes, as to cause catarrhal disease and dyspepsia. They tend to weaken digestion by calling for an undue secretion of digestive juices, which, if prolonged, tires out the glands.

The use of salts is discussed on pages 34–37.

A reasonable amount of condiments such as pepper, salt, nutmeg, cloves, allspice, sage, thyme, ginger, mustard, cinnamon, mace, horseradish, vanilla, dill, etc., may be used as appetizers, because the pleasing thought of them may incite the flow of gastric juice; but they should not be used to excess.

The taste is undoubtedly a cultivated one, and should not be encouraged in children. The child rarely cares for condiments and it is better that he continue to relish his food in its natural flavor.

If beef tea, which so soon becomes distasteful to the sick, is flavored with different savory or aromatic substances, as parsley, sage, or mint, it is taken with greater relish.

Mustard, so commonly used with cold ham or other meat and in salad dressing, is sometimes of benefit in stimulating the appetite, but when used in large quantities, or continuously, it may irritate the stomach. This irritant quality may be used to advantage, when it is deemed necessary, as a counter-irritant on the skin, as in the well-known mustard plaster. A teaspoonful of mustard to a pint of lukewarm water is

an effectual emetic in cases in which it is necessary
or advisable to empty the stomach.

Capers, the flower buds of a bush grown in the
East, are put up in vinegar and used in sauces for
mutton.

Cinnamon, *nutmeg*, and *cloves* are useful in flavoring
foods; they take the flat taste from hot water and
impart a pleasant spiciness. Many can take milk
when flavored, and the slight amount necessary is in
no way injurious.

Preserved ginger is of value for flavoring cereal foods
and gruels for invalids.

Vinegar, used in excess, reduces the alkalinity of
the blood and aids in the destruction of red blood
corpuscles. It may thus produce anemia when used
in excess.

The acetic acid contained in *cider vinegar* aids the
softening of the muscle fiber of meat and thus facilitates its digestion. Because of its preservative qualities it is used in pickling vegetables and various kinds
of fish.

Vinegars made from grapes or other fruits are wholesome. Flavored vinegars, as tarragon, from the
herb of the same name, are useful as appetizers.

Vinegars artificially made from commercial acids
are sometimes injurious.

Tomato Catsup, *Worcestershire*, and *Tabasco sauces*
are not harmful if used moderately and with due regard
to enhancing not destroying the flavor of the food
with which they are used.

PRESERVATION OF FOODS

This subject is of ever-growing importance. The
study of the preservation of foods has added much to

the store of human knowledge. By this means it is possible for those living in districts remote from the supply, those who cannot afford to buy them fresh, and those who have no cellars in which to store them, to have vegetables and fruits at all seasons of the year.

Nutritious foods can be prepared in such small bulk and of such excellent keeping quality that explorers, whether to the arctics or the tropics, can be kept in first-class physical condition, enabled to withstand fatigue, and be removed to long distances from the base of supplies without great hardship.

The decomposition of food is occasioned by bacterial action. Air is necessary to the growth of bacteria. If the air is excluded the ordinary bacteria are prevented from exerting their deleterious action.

Heat, as in canning, prevents the formation of bacterial products.

Cold, in refrigeration, by inhibiting bacterial activity is also an excellent preservative.

Other methods in use are smoking, salting, drying, sterilizing, various antiseptics, and the exclusion of the air, as in coating eggs or meat for transportation to other countries.

Eggs are preserved for a long period by excluding the air, which otherwise penetrates the shell. A solution of water glass (silicate of sodium), dry oats or salt are used for this purpose.

All food intended for preservation should be kept in a clean, cool, dry, dark place.

Drying, cooking, and sealing from the air will preserve some meats and fruits, while others require such preservatives as sugar, vinegar, and salt. The preservative in cider vinegar is acetic acid, in wine vinegar tartaric acid.

All preservatives which are actual foods, such as sugar, salt, and vinegar, are to be recommended, but the use of antiseptic preservatives, such as salicylic acid, formaldehyd, boracic acid, alum, sulphur, and benzoate of soda, all of which have been used by many canning merchants, is fraught with danger. By the efforts of the United States Department of Agriculture the use of such preservatives has been largely done away with by the most reliable packers and canners. However, unscrupulous dealers may use this means of disguising fruits and vegetables not in good condition.

There can be no doubt, that, whenever possible, the best method is for the housewife to preserve her own food by drying, canning, preserving, and pickling, with fruits and vegetables which she knows are fresh. This, however, is not always practicable.

Since economy in food lies in obtaining the greatest amount of nutriment for the least money, the preparation of simple foods in the home, with care that no more is furnished for consumption than the system requires, is the truest economy.

More brands of prepared food are not so much needed as purity of elements in their natural state.

In the effort to emphasize the importance of pure food in amount and quality, pure air and pure water must not be overlooked. Much infection is carried by these two elements.

POISONING FROM FOOD

Owing to the careful inspection given to various preparations of foods and the education of the people on the dangers attending the eating of underripe, overripe, or fermenting fruits and vegetables, or de-

8

composing canned meats or other foods, cases of poisoning from food are not so numerous as formerly.

One still reads, however, of illnesses and even fatalities in those who have, at some gathering, partaken of potted or canned meats, or ice-cream made from impure milk.

Imperfect sterilization allows the micro-organisms, everywhere present in the atmosphere, to multiply and produce their toxins.

Any food contained in a can which shows a suspicious bulging in top or sides (not a dent caused by handling) should be unhesitatingly rejected, for fermentation has developed gases, which, in trying to escape, have caused the bulging. Though the practice is less common than formerly, some grocers offer these bulging cans for sale at less prices and they are thus purchased by those who look for bargains in foods instead of for quality.

Sometimes the foods have not advanced to a stage in which the poisonous products are manifested; but in the intestinal canal the germs contained in these foods manufacture toxins which are readily absorbed and produce the severe disturbances noted in cases of ptomain poisoning.

The liver, which has been styled the "watchdog of the body," has a special power to destroy many of the toxins contained in the food material passing through it, and it is due to this fact that many deleterious substances, taken with the food, are neutralized and their poisons rendered harmless to the system. When the liver is disordered, this important function may be hindered, or cease to be active. Therefore, the importance may be readily seen of keeping the liver in a vigorous condition by means of exercises which will send an active circulation through it and keep the nerves controlling it in perfect functioning order.

Ptomain poisoning results most often from tainted meat, milk, and fish. Putrefactive processes may have begun in meat, which is thus rendered "high," but if it is thoroughly cooked the poisons may be made inert. Many enjoy the flavor of such meat. The Eskimos, as is well known, will cache a seal or other animal against a time when food is less plentiful and after months, perhaps, will eat it with relish and without harm, though it cannot be touched by people with less hearty appetites. Old eggs, eaten as a luxury by the Chinese, and the fermented fish used by other races are familiar examples of tainted foods.

The sale of "bob" veal, or the flesh of very young calves, has been prohibited because in many people its ready decomposition causes active diarrhea.

The process of smoking various meats affects materially only the outside portion, the inner may furnish a suitable bed for the development of germs. Great care should be exercised and thorough inspection made of any meat which is eaten raw, as dried beef, or any pork product.

Ice-cream, as made in the home, is usually innocuous, but when it is made in factories, unless care is exercised to keep containers clean and sterilized, the cream or milk may become infected from careless handling, either before or after it reaches the factory—particularly in warm weather. Toxins which cause serious and often fatal poisoning develop. Many such cases have resulted from the free eating of infected ice-cream at picnics or other social gatherings.

One should guard against overripe cheese, though

cheese of any kind acts as a poison with some people. Cases of severe intestinal disturbance may occur in those who are unable to eat certain articles of food, as strawberries, lobsters, or oysters; these attacks should be carefully distinguished from cases of true poisoning.

Sometimes, however, particularly in the case of fish or oysters which have been frozen, unless they are eaten immediately after they have been thawed, toxins develop which cause severe constitutional disturbance, particularly of the nervous system. These toxins do not seem to affect the gastro-intestinal tract so markedly. Infected shellfish, particularly mussels, have caused death in two hours by their effect on the nervous system.

Many fish after being smoked are eaten raw, and if the ptomains have begun to develop, poisoning follows.

Care must be taken in purchasing fish for the table that the flesh is firm and the odor absolutely without taint.

Meat or fish may become toxic to the system through substances eaten by the animal or by its own physical condition at the time it is killed. Fish and oysters, therefore, are not eaten during the spawning season.

Cow's milk may be made obnoxious by substances on which the cow feeds. Wild garlic when eaten by the cow imparts a nauseous taste to the milk.

The flesh from diseased animals slaughtered and sold for food has occasioned violent sickness. Government inspection, however, has greatly lessened the dangers from this source.

Unripe or overripe vegetables and fruit may occasion severe vomiting and diarrhea.

Moldy flour contains a substance which may cause poisoning.

Rye may have a parasite fungus called ergot and if flour is made from rye contaminated with this growth, a form of poisoning called "ergotism" may result. It takes some time and a prolonged use of the flour to cause untoward symptoms.

Pellagra, which has been giving the southern states so much trouble, was thought to be caused by the use of spoiled corn meal. It is now thought to be due to the disturbed nutrition following too monotonous and unbalanced a diet. The excessive use of corn-meal breads with their heating qualities and the irritation of the intestinal canal may be an accessory factor.

A food which is so universally used as milk should be surrounded with every safeguard possible by rigid inspection from producer to consumer, as many infective epidemics have been traced directly to a careless or infected handler of this product. Tuberculosis and typhoid fever germs, diphtheria and scarlet fever may all be communicated by this means. Live typhoid bacilli have been found in acid buttermilk. Infected water used in washing the cans will infect the milk.

Other poisoning may occur by the tin or lead in the inside of cans being dissolved off by the acids in fruits or vegetables. This is more likely to occur when the cans of fruit have been kept for a long time. Housekeepers, who use tin cans, should not put up more fruit than will supply the family for the season.

Tomatoes, asparagus, strawberries, and apricots are especially liable to dissolve the tin from the can.

Food should be emptied from the can as soon as it

is opened, as the action of the air hastens deterioration. No cooked fruit should be allowed to stand in a tin saucepan or other vessel. It should be emptied as soon as the cooking process is complete.

When a can of fruit, vegetables, or meat is opened, if the interior of the can is even partially black, it is safe to reject the contents. The tin in the food will be absorbed in the intestinal tract and may cause severe disturbance.

Large canners of fruit and vegetables, of the better quality, are now coating the inside of the can with an insoluble varnish which prevents the acids from acting on the tin.

The best canners are exceedingly careful and everything in their factories is scrupulously clean.

THE ADULTERATION OF FOOD

Laws against food adulteration have been enacted, but unscrupulous manufacturers find ways to evade them. On account of these laws, however, the practice is less general and manufacturers are beginning to take pride in putting up goods that pass the strictest inspection. The people, also, are being aroused, through the efforts of the pure-food propagandists, to the ill effects of adulterated foods both on the body and the pocketbook and are increasingly demanding that the foods they buy shall be pure and wholesome.

To lessen the cost of production, many foods are mixed with various substances before being marketed in order to increase the profits of the manufacturer or dealer. The contained substance may not be deleterious to health, but it may lessen the value of the article as a food.

Among foods which may be so adulterated are

jellies, jams and marmalades, catsups and pickles of all varieties, baking powder, butter, spices, coffee, corn-starch, mincemeat, vinegar, syrups, sugar, honey, lard, and flour.

Various adulterants which are used are: wood alcohol (a poison) in flavoring extracts; vinegar made from various acids and colored to imitate cider vinegar; rice flour and wheat flour used in ground spices; kaolin and coloring matter used in candies; paraffin in gum drops; glucose artificially flavored as maple syrup; cotton-seed oil sold as olive oil; starch and sugar in powdered cocoa and in chocolate; chicory, sugar, and pea meal in ground coffee; artificial coffee beans made of starch, molasses, and chicory; alum and ammonia in baking powders; artificial coloring of canned peas, beans, and catsups, butter, cheese, milk, and cream.

It must be said, in justice, however, that house-wives are responsible for many of these productions. Dealers who would be glad to sell only pure articles say that "the trade won't have them."

Many insist on a highly colored cheese, thinking that the color denotes greater richness, whereas a little reasoning would show them that the richest old cheeses are pale in color, the deeper color of the cheese being due to the addition of coloring matter to the curd. While the coloring matter is not deleterious, the color is no evidence of richness.

Highly colored green pickles, beans, and peas, should not be used. Pickles which are hard and crisp are usually made so by alum.

Brilliant red catsup is in demand, though the pure variety is known by its darker and not so attractive hue.

High coloring in any canned fruit or vegetable is usually an indication that dye stuffs have been used to produce it.

Fruit jams which are of nondescript color or pale when pure are colored artificially because the ordinary purchaser demands a pretty product.

Through the vigilance of the food inspectors of the boards of health, and because of some vigorous prosecutions, the adulteration of the people's food is, however, not so easy and profitable an occupation as formerly.

The Bulletins of the Department of Agriculture furnish a mine of wealth in the gaining of knowledge of various foods and their preparation, and may be had free on application to this Department at Washington.

HEAT AND ENERGY

The second use of foods, as mentioned before, is to furnish heat and energy for the work of the body. Heat and energy are produced *automatically* by the action of the heart, the movement of the lungs in breathing, and by muscular activity through the digestion, absorption, and assimilation of food elements, and through the activity in tearing down and eliminating waste. They are produced *consciously* by muscular activity in exercise.

Just as any engine requires fuel, water, and air to create the force necessary to run the machinery, so does the human engine require fuel, air, and water.

The fuel for an engine consists of coal, wood, or oil. As these are brought in combination with oxygen, combustion or oxidation takes place, liberating heat and setting the engine in motion.

The amount of energy or force given off by an engine should exactly equal the amount of latent energy provided in the fuel. Much of this energy is commercially lost, since much of the latent force in fuel is not fully liberated, some passing off in the smoke, while some may remain in the cinders.

The amount of heat and energy generated by the body equals the amount of latent energy released by the burning of food material during oxidation.

The carbohydrates and fats constitute the most of the fuel.

The body cells are constantly surrounded by the lymph which contains the food material—the protein, the carbohydrate, and the fat.

The lymph carries all of the food elements, therefore the protein, the fat, and the carbohydrate reach the tissues at the same time. If the fat and carbohydrate predominate, their excess serves to keep a portion of the protein away from the cells. The cells can use carbohydrate more easily than fat, so the surplus amount of carbohydrate is first used to produce energy. This spares the protein which is held in reserve for tissue repair, and the fat, being least readily used, is stored.

When the carbohydrates and fats are not supplied, or when the system fails for any reason to appropriate those eaten to its use, the protein is used for heat and energy instead of being used for tissue building. If the demand, either in mental or physical energy, exceeds the daily supply for long, the body becomes lean.

In order, therefore, to maintain a perfect equilibrium the supply of protein, carbohydrate, and fat should bear the proper relation, any excess at one time being equalized at another. If an overhearty meal is eaten the next should be light.

Fat is harder to burn than the starches and sugars so that they are acted on first as an economy of effort, and the fat is held in reserve until the carbohydrates are exhausted.

If one is cold, the quickest way to get warm is to generate more heat within by "turning on the draught," or, in other words, by *breathing in more oxygen.* If cold, one should depend more on the oxygen within than on extra clothing. So many people put on more clothing to conserve the body heat and forget to generate more heat by arousing the fires within. This is like covering a dying fire, instead of turning on the draught to create more combustion.

The carbon in the body is burned by being brought into contact with oxygen in the blood through exercise and full breathing, just as a fire is fanned to flame by bringing oxygen in contact with the fuel, by means of a draught of air. Keep all air away from a fire and it "dies out," it has exhausted the oxygen and no heat is produced; keep all air from within the body, by cessation of breathing, and it also dies.

A room is heated with difficulty if the air in it does not contain sufficient oxygen. Just so the body which is not constantly supplied with pure air generates very little heat. The effect of oxygen in the creation of heat is practically demonstrated by voluntary, rapid, deep breathing, completely filling the lungs with air, while out in the cold. The body will become quickly warmed on the coldest day by this practice.

Ten to twelve deep breaths in succession "turn on the draught" inside and create combustion (heat), just as opening the draught to a stove by causing

more air to circulate within it increases combustion
or heat.

Remember that heat is the result of combustion—
the more rapid the combustion in the body, caused
by oxygen breathed in through the lungs, the greater
the heat.

Just as much heat is created when fat is burned
in the body as when it is burned outside of the body.

The heat from "burning" wood is produced by the
union of the oxygen from the air with hydrogen and
carbon, forming carbon dioxid and water.

The light in the burning of wood is caused by the
rapid combustion. Combustion occurs within the
body more slowly, hence no light is produced.

The exact process by which the potential energy
latent in food is converted into heat and energy is
not known. It is partly released during the digestive
process, through the chemical action produced when
the elements of the food come into contact with oxygen and with the digestive juices. This combustion
gives to the digestive organs the necessary warmth
to enable them to do effective work. A certain
amount of heat is necessary for the chemical changes,
and digestive juices flow more freely when the body
is warm. Heat is necessary, also, to aid the peristaltic
movements of the digestive organs.

It has been estimated that about one-sixth of the
heat liberated evaporates through the skin, the lungs,
and the excreta, while five-sixths is required to maintain the body heat.

If the digestive forces are not working perfectly
and if the food is not properly prepared, some of the
fuel is not utilized. But, in normal conditions, if
the food is supplied in proportion to the energy re-

quired, the heat and energy given off should exactly equal the latent heat and energy consumed.   If more food is taken than is necessary to produce heat and energy, the excess of material is stored and if the excess continues the bodily machinery may be clogged. The relief lies in consuming the excess through exercise.   More oxygen is required to put the excess in condition for use, and the extra amount of oxygen is gained by means of the deep breathing occasioned by exercise.

It is to be noted, also, that no force within the body is lost.   In the very process of the removal of waste, heat and energy are created, so that the parts no longer needed are utilized by the system, while they are being removed from it.   Here is a lesson in economy of force.

A small portion of the heat of the body is gained from the sun or from artificial heat, but by far the greater part is generated within the body.

As mentioned before, the fuel for the body consists of *fats, starches, and sugars*, which, in combination with oxygen, create force.

From the foregoing, it follows that the fuel value of any food depends on the amount of fats, starches, and sugars it contains.

The chemical combination of oxygen with food elements and with the body tissue is known as *oxidation*.   It is this chemical action of the oxygen on the food and on the tissues which produces heat and energy, either in muscle, gland, or nerve.   This energy, in the muscle, expresses itself in movement; in the gland, in chemical action, and in the nervous system, by activity of brain or nerve centers.   The nervous energy is closely allied to electrical force.

Nature provides for a reserve of heat and energy, above the immediate needs, by storing a supply of heat-producing material which is utilized whenever the daily supply is insufficient or is lacking. Many hibernating animals store up sufficient fat in summer to provide heat for the entire winter. This fat would not last throughout the winter, however, were the animal active. Many individuals carry sufficient fat to supply all of their needs for months, even though all fat-building elements were omitted from the diet.

The fact that more oxygen is required for combustion of fat than of starches and sugars is important for those who wish to call on the fats stored within the body for daily heat and energy and thus reduce in weight.

If sufficient starches, sugars, and fats are not consumed in the body to supply the daily heat and energy released by exercise, the body calls on the reserve store in the tissues. If much fat or carbohydrates are consumed in the daily food this will be oxidized before the fat stored in the muscular tissue is called on.

The scientific reduction of weight, therefore, lies in the regulation of the daily consumption of starches, sugars, and fats, and the oxidation of more of these substances through an increase in the daily exercise.

Deep breathing of pure air should accompany all exercises to supply sufficient oxygen for combustion or oxidation.

In warm weather little fat is needed for fuel, and Nature provides fresh green vegetables to replace the root vegetables of the cold weather, which, consisting largely of starches and sugars, are readily converted into heat.

In cold weather, especially in high altitudes or latitudes, more fuel foods are required to keep the body warm and more fat is eaten.

It must be remembered that anything which creates a greater activity of the tissues, such as muscular exercise, liberates a greater amount of heat. The reverse is also true. A decrease in the amount of muscular movement means a decrease in the liberation of heat. During exercise, a large amount of carbohydrates and fats are released by the movements and oxidized; the liberated heat is carried to all parts of the system and the temperature is raised.

Food in the alimentary canal causes an activity in the glands of the digestive organs maintaining their temperature.

Of course, while digestion and muscular activity are at their height, the body temperature is highest. The temperature, as a rule, decreases from about six at night until four or five in the morning, when it is usually at its ebb. This is a point of importance. A degree or two of increase in temperature, above normal, if recorded about six at night, is not, in most conditions, considered alarming by the physician.

Anything which causes an increase in heat radiation, as perspiration, lowers the temperature, and the open pores of the skin are valuable aids in equalizing the body heat. A person who perspires freely does not suffer with heat during excessive exercise, as does one whose pores are closed.

Diuretic foods and beverages, such as water and fruits (melons, lemons, oranges, grapefruit, etc.), which increase the activity of the skin and the kidneys, also tend to lower the body temperature.

One ready means of regulating the body heat is the

bath. If one takes a hot bath, the temperature is
materially raised by the artificial heat, but there is a
recompense in the increase of heat radiation from
the skin and the reaction is cooling. If one takes
a cold bath, the immediate effect is cooling, but the
activity set up within, to create a reaction, soon
heats the body to a greater degree than before the
bath.

The best way to increase the evaporation and thus
decrease the temperature of the body is by a tepid
shower or a tepid sponge. The tepid water will not
create a strong reaction, and it will cause a decrease
in temperature. Thus, for fever patients or on a
warm day, the tepid shower or sponge is commended;
for a cold day, or for the individual whose circulation
is sluggish, the cold bath, followed by friction, is
desirable. When the vitality is low, so that reaction
is slow or chilly feelings persist, the bath must be
tempered and greater friction used.

The generation of heat is also increased by solid
foods that require more than normal activity on the
part of the digestive organs. For this reason the
food given fever patients should be that most easily
digested and should be reduced in quantity. Liquid
or semi-liquid foods are best.

While the elements of the food are being oxidized,
the latent (potential) energy released by the oxygen
creates mental and physical force and keeps active
the metabolic changing of food into tissues and cells,
also the changing of cells and tissues into waste.

Scientists have measured the energy latent in food
material, also the amount of heat given off in the
oxidation of a given quantity of waste. The unit
of measurement is the *calorie*—the amount of heat

which will raise one pound of water 4 degrees Fahrenheit.

The fuel value of any food denotes the total number of calories which may be derived from a pound of that food if it be completely oxidized in the body.

C. F. Langworthy gives the fuel value of proteins, fats, and carbohydrates as follows:

1 pound of protein yields..................... 1860 calories
1   "   " fats   " 4220   "
1   "   " carbohydrates yields.............. 1860   "

That is, according to fuel value—the capacity of the nutrients for yielding heat and mechanical power— a pound of the protein of lean meat or egg albumen just about equals a pound of starch or sugar, and about two pounds of these would about equal a pound of the fat of meat or of the body fat.

The calculation has been made, based on experiments, that one who does no muscular work needs only an amount of food which will produce 2700 calories. One doing light muscular work needs 3000 calories. An individual doing moderately heavy work should take 3500 calories, while heavy muscular work takes 4500 calories.

One hundred grams of protein food, however, gives only fifteen per cent. of the amount of energy required. About 500 grams of carbohydrate and 50 grams of fat are needed to make up the 3000 calories which must be furnished by the daily supply of food for one doing light muscular work.

The brain worker, who is using brain tissue more rapidly than the day laborer, should have a diet equally as rich in protein, though less fat and carbohydrates are needed.

It has been estimated that an ordinary man on full diet excretes about twenty grams (about five-eighths of an ounce) of nitrogen a day. As protein material contains about sixteen per cent. of nitrogen, such an individual needs to take about 120 grams of protein a day to supply the nitrogen needs of the body. Because of its need for protein, the body does not store it.

A day laborer needs 0.28 of a pound of protein a day with enough fat and carbohydrate to give a fuel value of 3500 calories. A professional man requires 0.25 ($\frac{1}{4}$) of a pound of protein a day. Much more than this is usually taken. This means from $\frac{1}{3}$ to $\frac{1}{2}$ a pound of lean meat.

Nothing is lost in Nature's distribution of force and energy. Everything accomplished in life, either in the physical handling of material, the brain work in planning the constructions, the mental movements of thought in art, literature, or science, are all representatives of the heat and energy released from the body, and every man and woman should endeavor to make the body yield as large an income as possible in the expression of this energy. In order that it may do so, it must be used with intelligence, just as any other great machine must be used intelligently; it must be fed, exercised, and rested judiciously.

9

CHAPTER V

THE work of the body never stops. If it is to be kept in thorough working order its tissues must be rebuilt as incessantly as they are torn down in the process of producing heat and energy. These chemical changes are called collectively *metabolism*.

They are divided into two groups: the chemical process of building up complex substances from simple ones is known as *anabolism;* the chemical process of oxidizing and breaking down the complex substances into simple ones, so that they are in a state to be excreted, is called *catabolism*. While the process of oxidation in catabolism is going on, heat and energy are set free. Many of the chemical changes in the body are catabolic in character. This work never ceases—even in sleep.

It is not enough that the proper foods be furnished the body in kind and quantity. The essential thing is that the system be kept in condition to *assimilate* the foods to its needs and to promptly eliminate the waste. Few people assimilate all of the foods eaten.

By *assimilation* is meant the process by which food-stuffs are made soluble and diffusible, so that they can pass into the blood; also, the metabolic activity by which the food is converted into cells and tissues.

Truly the body is a busy workshop. Think of the billions on billions of cells being formed and destroyed every instant in the liberation of heat and force! Think, also, of the necessity of perfect circulation to bring sufficient blood to the lungs, that it may gather the oxygen and carry it, without pausing for rest, to every tissue of the body! Even in sleep this stream continues incessantly.

There is also a great lesson here in the law of supply and demand. When the body is at mental or muscular work, the potential energy liberated leaves through muscle or brain, as energy, and is expressed in the result of the work. When the body is at rest, energy leaves it as heat (excepting such part as is necessary to carry on metabolism, circulation, etc.).

If much muscular energy is called for, a deep, full breath is instinctively drawn to supply the oxygen necessary for the added force.

If strong mental work is required, attention should be given to exercise and deep breathing, that the blood may carry off the waste liberated by brain activity. The difficulty is that in doing close mental work, the body is too frequently bent over a desk in such a manner as to restrict the action of the lungs; thus, the brain worker, in order to continue strong mental work, must often go into the open air, as he says, "to rest his brain," but in reality to obtain the oxygen needed to put the waste, liberated by brain energy, in condition to be carried away. The supply of blood has been called on for the brain work; the poor circulation through the body has allowed an excess of carbon dioxid to accumulate and the condition of the body designated as "tired" has resulted. Until the necessary oxygen has been supplied, the brain and body are not balanced, not "rested."

In its conversion into tissue, heat, energy, and waste, the importance of the chemical exceeds that of the mechanical action of digestion, absorption, assimilation, and elimination; yet the chemical changes are aided by the mechanical.

Nature provides against ignorance of the amount of supply necessary, by enabling the system to carry off a limited amount of surplus food above the bodily requirements. Her capacity in this regard is limited and varies with each individual. Therefore common sense is required in deciding for oneself the amount of food which will aid, and not hinder Nature in her processes.

Without doubt many eat more food than the system requires, and when it is overloaded they do not take the pains to burn up and eliminate the excess through exercise and oxygen.

On the other hand, this theory of overeating has been so long discussed that many have not eaten sufficient food and their bodies are undernourished. Many, also, from lack of exercise, hence lack of demand of the body for food, have supposed this lack of appetite to be Nature's call "Enough"; inertia has resulted and waste remains in the body. They have failed to exercise sufficiently to create a demand for food. It is thus undernourished because sufficient new building material has not been supplied. The relief from this condition is exercise and deep breathing so that Nature removes the waste and calls for fresh building material.

Many others, through mental and physical activity, burn up much fuel and the result is the body does not store up sufficient fat for a reserve, or for beauty and comfort. The nerves require a certain amount of fat for their protection. People of this type should take a more full and sometimes a more varied diet, particularly more liquid, and should not fail in daily exercise and deep breathing.

Each individual should know, approximately, the chemical constituents and the proportion of these constituents in normal blood, because from the elements in the blood, the tissues are constructed. If certain elements are lacking, the foods containing these elements in largest proportions should be supplied until the blood no longer shows the deficiency. This is Nature's method of correction. The variations in the blood can be known only by chemical analyses and until physicians have access to chemical laboratories the giving of drugs cannot be a science.

Each meal, or each day's food, may not contain the amount of protein or of fuel ingredients necessary for that day's work and resupply, but the body is continually storing material, and this reserve is constantly being drawn on to provide any element which may be lacking in that day's supply. Thus, an excess or a deficiency one day may be adjusted the next. Healthful nourishment requires that the balance, as a whole, be kept and that a deficiency or oversupply be not continued for too long.

The distinct steps in anabolism and the effect of oxygen on assimilation are discussed in the following pages.

DIGESTION

Any discussion of the digestibility of foods must be general, because food which agrees with one may disagree with another, and a food which disagrees with one at a particular time may entirely agree with him at some other time according to the condition of his system.   Therefore, before one passes on the adaptability of a food to his system, he should know that this food agrees or disagrees with him under various conditions.

The chances are that the food is right but that the attitude of mind and the condition of the body are abnormal.

The digestibility of food depends largely on the physical condition of the individual, because the amount of digestive juices poured into the alimentary canal is influenced by this condition, particularly by the condition of the nerves.   If sufficient juices, in proper proportions, are not poured into the digestive tract, the foodstuffs are not made soluble for absorption.

Digestion is practically synonymous with solution —all solid foods must be reduced to a liquid state by means of the digestive juices and water before they can pass through the walls of the stomach and intestines and enter the blood.

Each individual should learn to like the foods containing the nutrient elements which experience and blood tests have shown to be lacking in his case.

Yet while it is true that in most cases the aversion to a particular food is largely mental, there are kinds of food which, to certain individuals, according to the chemical composition of the body, act as actual poisons, e. g., strawberries, cheese, or coffee.

· The question of likes and of dislikes in foods, is largely habit, and one can learn to like almost any food, if one really has the desire to do so.

When the habit has been formed of discriminating too much in the food, of discarding this food or that, because at some time it has disagreed, due to the particular condition at the time, the mind approaches the table in a pessimistic attitude and the saliva and the gastric juices are retarded in their flow.

When one is exercising freely, so that the muscular and mucous coats of the digestive system are strong, the body will handle foods which, during sedentary habits, it would not digest.

Much indigestion is due to mental apathy. The mind often needs arousing to an interest in something.

Such an individual needs to know that one of the hardest things for the members of his family is to live day by day with one who maintains an attitude of mental depression, and he should stir himself for "his stomach's sake," as well as for the sake of his family, to a cheerful interest in something. He should let go his grudge and ride a hobby, if it is a cheerful one, and ride it hard.

It may be well, here, to trace, briefly, the progress of the food through the digestive tract and the action of the juices and the ferments on it.[1]

The food in the mouth is mixed with saliva, which begins the dissolution of the starches.

Salivary Digestion

The saliva consists of about 99.5 per cent. water

---

[1] For a knowledge of the structure and function of the mucous lining of the stomach and intestines, and of the tributary glands, such as the liver and pancreas, which is important to a thorough understanding of digestion, the reader is referred to *Let's Be Healthy*, of this series. In this will be found a study of the secretion of digestive juices, the conditions favoring normal secretions, etc.

and 0.5 per cent. solids. The solids consist of ptyalin, sodium chlorid, sodium carbonate, mucus, and epithelium. Ptyalin, the most important of these, is the active digestive agent; the mucus lubricates the masticated food; the sodium carbonate insures the alkalinity of the food, and the water dissolves the food that the juices may more readily reach and act on each particle.

The starches are the only foods whose chemical digestion is begun in the mouth. They are first broken up by the ptyalin into dextrin and then into the more simple sugar, known as maltose.[1]

It is important that sufficient saliva be mixed with the food through mastication, because unless the digestion of the starches is begun by the saliva, either in the mouth or after it is swallowed, they are not acted on until they reach the small intestine, consequently their digestion is unduly delayed. The pancreatic juice must then do more than its normal work of digestion.

The saliva flows into the mouth, more or less, at all times, but more copiously during mastication.

The movement of the jaws in chewing incites its flow and when starches are not well digested, gum chewing, in moderation, though not a refined habit, is beneficial.

The evident purpose of the saliva when food is not present is to keep the lining of the mouth moist

Salivary digestion is carried on in the stomach until the food becomes thoroughly mixed with the gastric

---

[1] Hereafter, in speaking of sugar, after it has been absorbed into the blood, the reader will bear in mind that the term refers not only to digested sugar, consumed as such, but also to digested starches (maltose).

juice, which, being acid, inhibits the action of the ptyalin.

The thorough and regular cleansing of the teeth is an important aid to digestion. Food products allowed to remain about the teeth ferment, rendering the mouth acid. When the mouth is acid, the alkaline saliva does not secrete in sufficient amount and the mouth is more or less dry.

The mouth is acid in rheumatism and allied conditions and the saliva may be thick and ropy so that it does not moisten the food properly. On the other hand the flow of saliva may be too free, the ptyalin is then too much diluted to promptly act on the food. This may result from overstimulation of the salivary glands occasioned by the excessive chewing of gum, or tobacco. These excesses also carry too much air into the stomach, resulting in flatulence.

The flow of saliva is controlled, largely, by nerves centering in the medulla oblongata. The sight of food, pleasingly served, or even the thought of food which one likes, will increase the flow. This is one instance of the control of thought over digestion, and the importance of forming the habit of cultivating a taste for all kinds of food is apparent. The stronger the relish for the food, and the more thoroughly it is masticated and mixed with the saliva, the more perfectly will the first step in digestion be accomplished.

Thorough mastication is important, not only because the chemical action on the starch molecules is facilitated by the softening and mixing with the saliva, but also because thorough mastication tends to prevent overeating—the appetite is more quickly satisfied when the food is well masticated.

Cool water encourages the flow of saliva and for this reason should be drunk before meals, particularly when digestion is weak. It may be taken at rest periods during the meal. (See page 31.)

The relation of the mouth and nasal

The Mouth and Nasal Passages passages to the digestive processes is seldom considered by the average individual. Their importance to the growing child is being recognized by the examination of school children which is now being made a part of the health program in many of our cities. Their importance to the adult is no less.

Food particles allowed to remain around the teeth, or in the cavities of decayed teeth, incite bacterial action. With the next meal these bacteria are swallowed and cause fermentation of the food, occasioning indigestion, and possibly, dyspepsia.

Decayed or missing teeth, swollen gums, or pyorrhea, interfere with proper mastication of food, hence it does not receive the thorough salivary moistening necessary; the starches pass practically unchanged into the stomach and small intestine, overburdening these organs.

Catarrh of the nasal passages, with the constant swallowing of germ-filled secretions, carries morbid products into the stomach, coating the glands with mucus, often infecting them; it may also occasion a catarrhal condition of that organ.

If, from any cause, the saliva becomes acid, dryness of the mouth results and desire for food is lessened or absent. Diseases of the salivary glands may render these necessary secretions unfit to perform their work.

In illness the mouth often drops open from weakness, producing the same condition of dryness. The mouth, in illness, is too often neglected by those in charge of the invalid.

Adenoids and enlarged turbinates in child or adult, narrowing the nasal passages and preventing the ingress of air, cause mouth breathing. The air dries the membranes and the tongue becomes swollen and cracks, interfering with proper mastication.

Adenoids should be removed, and any other condition which interferes with the proper function of the mouth should be remedied as soon as possible.

The mouth should be properly cleansed, the gums massaged, the teeth thoroughly brushed, back as well as front, defective teeth repaired or removed, abnormal growths eliminated, and the secretions kept abundant and healthy. Food well prepared in the mouth by thorough mastication satisfies hunger, renders more easy the work of the stomach and intestines, and aids in the general welfare of the system.

This too prevalent habit may aggravate the condition which it is supposed to cure. A slight indigestion appearing, gum is **Gum-chewing** often chewed to cause a fuller flow of saliva to aid digestion. If gum-chewing is indulged in to excess, however, the muscular movements overstimulate the salivary glands, eventually weakening them. Overuse of the chewing muscles and overexcitation of the nerves fatigue them and cause them to weaken. The sticky gum, adhering to fillings in the teeth, loosens them and furnishes a lodging place for food particles and bacteria.

The excess of saliva may render the gastric juice alkaline, inhibiting its action. Excess of air swal-

lowed with the saliva may cause flatulence or accumulation of gas in the stomach.

Lack of poise and nerve tension is increased by
excessive gum-chewing, resulting in fatigue of the
entire body. This lack of poise may be noted in any
public assembly, as the "movies," frequented by
gum-chewers.

The habit, as generally practiced, is not an inspiring
sight and should be discouraged.

Gum-chewing in moderation, for a few minutes
after a meal, may not do harm, but its indiscriminate use is to be deplored. Thorough mastication of food will serve to supply the necessary
saliva.

Exercise directed to the stomach and a more thorough circulation and elimination will do more for any
digestive derangement than the excessive practice of
chewing gum.

**Stomach
Digestion**
As the food enters the stomach, the
gastric juice pours out from the mucous
lining, very much as the saliva pours into
the mouth. Like the saliva, it consists of 99.5 per
cent. water and 0.5 per cent. solids. The solids of
the gastric juice are pepsin, rennin, hydrochloric acid,
and mucus.

The *mucus* serves to lubricate the food as in the
saliva. It perhaps also aids to prevent the digestion
of the mucous lining of the stomach.

The *hydrochloric acid* and the *pepsin* cause the
principal chemical changes in the food while in the
stomach. They act only on the proteins. The
hydrochloric acid must be present before the pepsin
can act, as only in an acid medium can pepsin dissolve

the proteins.   It is also of an antiseptic nature and hinders or prevents the decomposition of food.

The *rennin* ferment precipitates the casein.

The only digestion of starches in the stomach is that continued by the saliva.

Gastric juice begins to flow into the stomach soon after eating, but normally it is not secreted in sufficient quantity to supersede salivary digestion for from twenty to forty-five minutes.

The result of gastric digestion of proteins is their conversion, first, into albumin, then into proteoses, and, lastly, into peptone, which is protein in a more simple, soluble, and diffusible form.   In the form of peptone, the proteins are in condition to be absorbed.

If the food has been properly cooked and masticated, gastric digestion will be completed in from one and one-half to three hours.   If not properly cooked and masticated, the stomach digestion may continue from one to two hours longer.   It should, however, be completed in three hours.

It will be seen that the evening meal is ordinarily digested before sleep, as one does not retire for from three to five hours after eating.

If, through imperfect mastication, or a disordered condition of the stomach, the digestion is not completed in about three hours, the food is likely to be retained in the stomach and by its weight may cause prolapsus of that organ if the supporting tissues are weak.   Fermentation may ensue and give rise to gases which may cause acute distress.

Animal foods, which are readily digested, remain in the stomach for a shorter time.   Meat, as a rule, is easily digested, because the digestive juices of the animal have converted the starches and sugars.   The white meat of chicken is digested in a shorter time than the red or the dark meat.

Corn, beets, peas, beans, etc., take about three and a half hours to digest; baked potatoes about two and a half hours.

Raw vegetables and fruits remain about the same length of time as potatoes.

Sugar is usually absorbed within an hour.

The cereals, if well cooked, take but two hours.

Coarse or badly masticated food, tough meats, unripe fruits, and much fat hinder digestion.

Undigested food passing into the intestine may fail to be acted on there and will sometimes produce diarrhea.

Fluids leave the stomach more rapidly than solids. Seven ounces of water entirely leaves the stomach in one and one-half hours, seven ounces of boiled milk in about two hours. Water and buttermilk almost immediately begin to pass out of the stomach; milk begins to pass out in about fifteen minutes.

The flow of gastric juice, as the flow of saliva, is governed by the nerves; the sight, taste, and smell of food, and the attitude of mind toward it, to a certain extent, regulate its flow.

After the food has accumulated, during the progress of a meal, the stomach begins a series of wave-like movements called peristaltic waves.[1] These waves propel the food through the length of the stomach towards its lower opening, known as the pyloric orifice. During this process the food is thoroughly mixed with the gastric juice.

During the early stages of digestion of solids, the sphincter muscles of the pylorus keep the lower open-

[1] See *Let's Be Healthy*, by Susanna Cocroft.

ing of the stomach closed, but, as digestion progresses, the pylorus gradually relaxes to let the digested, soluble portion of the food pass into the intestine. If the food still remains in a solid form, by reason of being improperly cooked or poorly masticated, as it touches the pylorus, these sphincter muscles, almost as if they were endowed with reasoning faculties, close, forcing the undigested mass back to be further acted on by the gastric juice—the solid mass is not allowed to pass until dissolved.

If the individual abuses the stomach and causes it to work overtime, it becomes exhausted and demands rest; it refuses to discharge the gastric juice in proper proportion; the peristaltic movements are weak; and food is not promptly or forcefully moved along the stomach and mixed with the gastric juice. This condition is termed indigestion.

The food passes from the stomach, through the pylorus into the small intestine. In this condition of partial digestion it is called chyme. **Intestinal Digestion**

The first twelve inches of the small intestine is known as the duodenum. In the duodenum the food is acted on by the pancreatic juice, the bile, and the intestinal juices. These juices act on proteins, fats, and carbohydrates. The bile acts on the fats, while the pancreatic and intestinal juices act on the proteins and the carbohydrates. The starches, or dextrin, not fully digested by the saliva, are changed to maltose and glucose, while the trypsin from the pancreatic juice, together with the intestinal juices, change into peptone the protein not fully digested in the stomach. The pancreatic juice also digests the starch found in raw fruits and in such raw vegetables as radishes and lettuce.

Fats are almost entirely digested in the small intestine. The presence of fat stimulates the flow of pancreatic juice, which, in turn, stimulates the flow of bile. For this reason, in some conditions, if the liver is sluggish, fatty foods in moderation are desirable. When bile is not present in sufficient amount the fatty foods ferment and cause gases and foul odors.

The fats are absorbed almost entirely in the small intestine—mostly in the duodenum. Some of the fat may be absorbed directly without undergoing the process of emulsification. Some oils, as paraffin oil, are not absorbed at all but act only as a lubricant of the intestines.

When the food enters the intestine its reaction is acid. Mixed with the bile, pancreatic and intestinal juices, which are alkaline, its reaction becomes alkaline.

The pancreatic juice splits up the fats into glycerin and fatty acids and enables the bile to exert its important emulsifying power. The bile markedly aids this action of the pancreatic juice though it has no fat-splitting power in itself.

Steapsin, another ferment of the pancreatic juice, acts on both fats and carbohydrates in either an acid or alkaline medium.

The sodium in the bile unites with the fatty acid, forming a soap which coats the tiny particles of fat and emulsifies them. The bile thus aids in the absorption of the fats. It also lubricates the intestinal mass, facilitating its passage through the entire length of the intestines. Thus it is a very potent agent in regulating the bowel movements.

A diminution in the flow of bile quickly expresses itself in constipation.

Fat and protein stimulate the activity of the liver, while starches, if taken in excess, incline to overload it.

The food is forced along the intestinal tract by peristaltic or muscular relaxation and contraction waves, as in the stomach. As it is so forced, the nutrient elements, after being put into condition for absorption, are taken up through the villi of the intestinal walls by the portal veins and the lacteals of the submucous lining.

A larger proportion of food is digested and absorbed than was formerly supposed, and the excretions from the intestines are, in many cases, made up almost entirely of refuse, and of the catabolic waste of the system. In an ordinary mixed diet, it is stated that about ninety-two per cent. of the proteins, ninety-five per cent. of the fats, and ninety-seven per cent. of the carbohydrates are retained by the body.

In digestion, it is of the utmost importance that the muscular, mucous, and submucous coats, and the secreting glands of the stomach and intestines be kept thoroughly strong and active, that the digestive juices may be freely poured out, the nutriment be freely absorbed, and the food be moved along the digestive tract. The strength of any organ is gained through the nutriment in the blood; therefore, daily exercise, which calls the blood freely to these organs is imperative. Daily exercise should be directed to the vital organs. A walk for exercise is not sufficient.

The greater part of the food is absorbed through the intestines, yet some proteins which have been fully digested by the gastric juice, and certain fats, particularly the fats

Absorption of Food

10

in milk, which are in a natural state of emulsion, may be absorbed through the walls of the stomach. However, the absorption through the stomach is small compared to that through the small intestine.

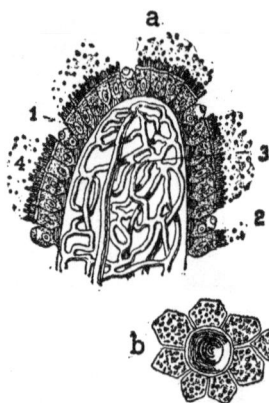

DIAGRAMMATIC REPRESENTA-
TION OF VILLUS.

a, I, cylindrical or "sucking" cells; 2, goblet cell; 3, capillaries; 4, food particles ready for absorption by the cells; *b*, cylindrical and goblet cells seen from above.—Adapted from LANDOIS.

The small intestine is peculiarly fitted for absorption. Its mucous lining is thrown up into folds to furnish a larger surface for this purpose. The folds hold the food as it passes toward the large intestine, until the villi have the opportunity to absorb it.

These transverse folds of the intestinal walls are called *valvulæ conniventes*.

The villi are tiny finger-like projections of the mucous lining of the intestines, which stand out of the lining somewhat as the nap on plush. They have been called "sucking" villi, because during the movements of the intestines they seem to suck in the liquid food.

As soon as the foodstuffs—proteins, carbohydrates, and fats—are put in an absorbable state called chyle, they are very promptly taken up by the villi.

If for any reason the chyle remains unabsorbed,

it is liable to be attacked by the bacteria always present in the intestines, and gases form.

The peptones, sugars, and saponified fats are rapidly absorbed, while the undigested portion, together with the unabsorbed water, the bile, mucus, and bacterial products, are passed through the ileocecal valve into the large intestine.

The mass passes up the ascending colon, on the right side of the abdomen, across the transverse, and down the descending colon, on the left side, losing, by absorption, the small amount of foodstuffs not absorbed in the stomach and small intestine. That the large intestine is to some extent adapted to absorption is shown by clinical experiments with patients who cannot retain food in the stomach, the food in such cases being given through rectal injections.

While water and salt are absorbed in both the stomach and small intestine, the larger part of the water passes into the large intestine, that it may assist the passage of the intestinal contents.

Water also stimulates peristaltic movements.

As the food is absorbed through the walls of the alimentary canal, it is picked up by the rootlets of the mesenteric veins and by the lymph channels— the latter through the abdominal cavity are called lacteals. Nearly all of the fats are absorbed through the lacteals. The whitish color given to the contents of the lacteals, by the saponified fats, gives rise to the term "lacteal."

Nearly all of the proteins and sugars pass through the mesenteric veins and the portal veins to the liver. Here the sugars are at once attacked by the liver cells and built up into glycogen as described on pages 151 and 159. A small portion of the proteins, how-

ever, do not go to the liver, but are passed directly
into the lymphatics and thus into the blood stream,
where they are again carried to the liver, and the urea
is separated.

To sum up, the larger part of the sugars, starches,
proteins, and fats is absorbed through the small intestine, a small amount being absorbed in the stomach and
a very little through the large intestine.   While some
water and salts are absorbed in the stomach and small
intestine, these are largely absorbed in the large
intestine.

**Economy
in Food**   It is economy to keep the digestive
organs and the circulation and tissues
strong, in order that all foods eaten may
yield returns, instead of hampering the activity of
the body.

The food which furnishes the most tissue-building
substance and yields the most heat and energy, with
the least refuse, is the economical food, provided it is
varied enough to meet the psychical needs as well as
the physical.

Whether or not a food is economical depends on
the degree to which it stimulates the activity of
the mind as well as the body.   Preparation and
serving here are as important as the material to be
served.

Economy in food is a question into which many
factors should enter.   A cheap food is not always an
economical food.   Amount and keeping qualities,
palatability, ripeness or unripeness, the age, habit,
and occupation of the partakers, all have their share
in the problem.

In the selection of food for any individual, the result to be gained from the food must be borne in mind. If one is doing heavy muscular work, more protein to rebuild tissue, as well as more carbohydrates and fats to produce energy, are required than if one's habits of work are sedentary.

In mental work, in which the brain is continually active, proteins are required to resupply the brain tissue, but the fats and carbohydrates may be lessened. If the brain is sufficiently active to use all of the fuel in brain energy one does not accumulate fat.

In sedentary occupations, which do not call for hard and continuous mental activity, the carbohydrates and fats, if taken in excess, are stored within the system, clogging it and producing torpid liver, constipation, and obesity.

In a study of tables of food values, in making up a dietary, the question should be to provide the largest quantity of nutriment at the lowest cost, with due attention to palatability and variety.

In the selection of meats, for instance, while beef steak may cost twice as much as beef stew, it must be borne in mind that beefsteak contains very little waste, and that it contains a large proportion of albuminoids, or the tissue-building proteins, while, in beef stew, bone and connective tissue predominate. A large proportion of the proteins obtained from the beef stew are gelatinoids and extractives—not the tissue-building albuminoids. (See page 56.)

In comparing the cheaper and the more expensive cuts in the same kind of beefsteak, however, the cheaper cuts often yield quite as much nutriment as the more expensive ones. Round steak is just as nourishing as porterhouse and cheaper, if one considers the greater number of helpings derived from a pound of round steak than from a pound of porterhouse.

For the aged or the invalid, however, the question of preparation will determine the relative economy.

CHAPTER VI

ORGANS AND CONDITIONS AFFECTING DIGESTION

THE purpose of this chapter is to show the work of other than the digestive organs in assimilation, construction, and elimination.

The *liver* is commonly called the chemical workshop of the body. The digested food is carried by the blood (portal veins) to the liver as soon as it is absorbed from the alimentary canal. As the food materials filter through the blood capillaries, between the liver cells, several substances are absorbed, particularly sugar, which is changed into the animal starch called *glycogen*. It is held in the liver for a few hours in this form and is then redigested and gradually given to the blood in the form of sugar.

While the conversion of the sugar is one prominent function of the liver, it also acts on the proteins—not as they are first passed through the liver in the blood, but as they are returned to the liver from the muscle tissue, partly oxidized and broken up into simpler products. The liver cells absorb and further oxidize and combine them into nitrogenous waste, which the kidneys throw off in urea.

The liver and the spleen also dissolve the pigment or coloring matter out of the red blood corpuscles. As these become useless, they are broken up in the liver and the spleen. The iron is retained by the liver cells and the remainder is thrown off in the bile.

The liver is on guard for all poisons which pass through it in the blood. The large part of these toxic substances are absorbed through the alimentary canal with the foodstuffs. Many of them are the result of the fermentation of foods which are not digested so promptly or so thoroughly as they should be, on account of an insufficient secretion of digestive juices, or on account of a failure to secrete them in normal proportions, due to inactivity of the stomach and intestines.

Nature thus supplies a guard to oxidize, or break down these poisons and make them harmless, so that normally they do not affect the nerves and the blood stream, and, through these, the entire system.

The necessity of correct habits of deep breathing will be readily seen here, because oxygen is required to break down the poisons as well as to oxidize the worn-out tissues.

One example of the action of the liver in rendering substances harmless, is its oxidation of *alcohol*. From one to three ounces of alcohol a day may be oxidized and made harmless in the liver, varying according to the individual and to the condition, at different times, in the same person. If the limit of one to three ounces is exceeded, the excess is not oxidized and intoxication results. This is the reason one may become intoxicated at one time when the same amount of liquor would not appreciably affect one at another.

The *muscles* play an important part in the use of foods. Most of the heat is generated in them by the action of the oxygen in the blood upon the sugar and fats, liberating their latent heat. This heat is liberated during every moment of the twenty-four hours whether one is asleep or awake. Of course, more is liberated during exercise, since the movement of the muscles sets all tissues into activity and the blood circulates more strongly, bringing a greater supply of oxygen to them.

It is always well during active exercise to stop frequently and fully inflate the *lungs*, not only to bring more oxygen to the blood, but to change the residual air and in the inflation to exercise the lung tissue more freely, bringing a better supply of nourishment to it. We forget that the lung tissue as well as every other tissue of the body needs exercise and a full supply of nourishment.

One should form the habit of breathing fully and deeply—otherwise the liberated carbon dioxid will cause an increased pressure throughout the blood stream, particularly about the heart and in the head. This pressure is relieved when the excess of carbon dioxid has been thrown off by the lungs. Much dull headache is due to the retention of carbon dioxid resulting from shallow breathing.

Nature makes the effort to throw off this excess of carbon dioxid by forcing one to breathe more rapidly while running or taking unusual exercise.

A certain amount of protein is constantly oxidized in muscular action also, being broken down into carbon dioxid, water, and a number of nitrogenous mid-products. The carbon dioxid and water are thrown off by the lungs, and the partially oxidized nitrogenous waste is carried to the liver, where it is further oxidized and prepared for excretion through the kidneys, lungs, skin, and intestines.

Through their stimulant action, the *nerves* aid in

oxidizing food materials. During periods of rest, food materials are also stored in the nerve cells. During nervous activity they are oxidized and carried away through the blood and the lymph. This oxidation of the food, stored in the nerves, creates nervous energy and heat.

The energy liberated by the nerves resembles electrical energy.

When one is continuously using an excess of nerve activity, all reserve food material, stored in the nerve cells, is used and the nerves become undernourished. The result is seen in neurasthenic conditions of various kinds.

The nerves as well as other tissues require protein to renew their substance as well as fats and carbohydrates for their energy.

The vasomotor nerves influence digestion to a marked extent by regulating the blood pressure in the digestive organs and the consequent rate of speed with which digestion and absorption take place. They speed up or slow down the movements of the alimentary canal, thus aiding and preventing the admixture of the food with the digestive juices. By acting on the glands, they aid or prevent the secretions from being formed and poured out. They thus materially affect digestion.

The vasomotor nerve centers are in the medulla oblongata.

The *lungs* absorb oxygen and eliminate carbon dioxid. They occasionally throw off a very little organic material.

The carbon dioxid is carried to the lungs from the tissues through the venous stream and diffused through the walls of capillaries in the lungs. The oxygen is absorbed in the thin air sacs in the capillary walls.

If the lungs are cramped by a faulty position of the body, by excess of fat, or by tight clothing, they cannot expand to their fullest extent. The blood is thus imperfectly aërated and oxygenized and is not freed of its waste. The lung tissue is imperfectly exercised, sufficient blood not being brought to the lung cells to insure their strength.

The cramping of the lungs is due largely to incorrect habits of standing and sitting.

The *kidneys* do not absorb as do the lungs, neither do they perform any anabolic work as does the liver, nor catabolic work as the muscles, nerves, and the liver. They simply throw off waste matter.

As the blood passes through them urea, uric acid, urates, sulphates, and sodium phosphates pass from it and with the water are thrown from the system; hence the kidneys are purifying organs, as are the lungs. The blood returning from the kidneys through the veins is pure, just as the blood in the pulmonary vein is pure, while that in the arteries to the kidneys is impure.

Interference with the action of the kidneys results in an excess of these substances in the blood and may produce a condition of intoxication known as uremic poisoning.

The *skin*, by pressure on the capillaries, controls, to some extent, their dilatation, and thus prevents an excessive loss of fluid. When a portion of the skin is removed by accident, as after burns, drops of moisture may be seen gathering on the denuded surface and may result in considerable loss if the denuded surface is large.

The skin is a protective covering. We are constantly surrounded with bacteria, dirt, etc., and the skin prevents their absorption.

It contains glands which secrete a fluid fat. This keeps the skin soft and flexible, preventing it from becoming too dry. The skin also prevents the underlying tissues from injury through abrasions or contact with foreign substances, as in various industries.

It also contains sweat glands, which throw off body waste in the form of salts and moisture in the perspiration; this helps to regulate the body heat and to aid in keeping the skin soft.

The kidneys and the skin are interdependent; if the kidneys are inactive the skin must throw off a larger quantity of waste and if the skin is inactive, or if for any reason its pores are closed, the kidneys become more active.

The skin also throws off carbon dioxid and, to a slight extent, it absorbs oxygen.

Besides digesting and absorbing food, the *intestines* eliminate waste.

In their work of elimination, they pass off all undigested matter. They also carry off bile pigment, bile salts, mucus, other decomposition products— also a little unabsorbed fat.

Coarse articles of food containing fibers which do not digest, such as the bran of grains and the coarser fibers of fruits and vegetables (much of their substances are not food in the strictest sense), are valuable, as they increase the peristaltic movements of the intestines and assist in carrying the waste excretions along their course.

The intestines also carry off the organic refuse which is produced by the chemical action of oxy-

gen.   This refuse consists of carbon dioxid and the
nitrogenous waste.

Combustion, or burning of fuel in any form (oxidation to release latent heat and energy), always leaves
a residue, and it is the work of the intestines to eliminate much of this refuse.   When coal is burned, gas,
smoke, ashes, and cinders constitute the waste; if
these were not allowed to escape or were not removed
from a stove the fire would soon go out—the smoke
and gas would smother it and the accumulation of
ashes would prevent the circulation of oxygen.

This is true in the body—the carbon dioxid not
being allowed to pass off would soon put out the fires
of life; it would poison the body and inhibit the action
of the nerves.   If the waste is not thrown from the
system we notice it in a feeling of lassitude, both
mental and physical.   If the nitrogenous waste (like
ashes and cinders) is not eliminated, one will die in
convulsions in a few days.

The absolute necessity of a free elimination of waste
will be readily seen.   If the engine is to do its work,
the engineer sees that it is kept perfectly clean—
otherwise it becomes clogged, works inefficiently, and
soon wears out.   The same is true in the body—
clogging in any part overworks and wears out other
parts dependent on the work of the defective one.

Constipation, or a failure of the intestines to eliminate the waste is a grave menace to the system.
The poisonous gases accumulating are absorbed by
the system.

The *blood* carries the digested food and the oxygen
to the various tissues and organs, which select from
among the nutrients offered to them the ones suited
to their growth and repair.

It is the universal medium of exchange.

It carries carbon dioxid to the lungs and the wastes of the tissues to the other eliminative organs.

It carries impure material to the purifying organs, and pure material away from them.

When it is lacking in quality or quantity the body suffers and if the lack continues the body dies.

Every organ contributes its share to the work of the blood and every organ takes from the blood some of its elements. If the blood pressure is too low, stagnation may occur. If it is too high an abnormal condition of the system results.

In fact, on the condition of the blood depends the effective working of the entire organism.

Constant effort then should be intelligently exerted to eat the proper foods, to exercise judiciously, to think healthful thoughts, to secure thorough elimination of waste in order that the whole body shall be fit for the work which its owner desires it to do.

SUMMARY

The processes which the food undergoes in digestion—conversion into condition to be absorbed by the body; in absorption through the walls of the intestines and stomach, and the metabolic processes which it undergoes in being converted into heat and energy and again broken down and eliminated as waste, are, in brief, as follows:

The Saliva begins the digestion of starches and sugars in the mouth, and continues this digestion for a time in the stomach.

The Stomach, when in normal condition, digests the proteins. If any proteins fail of digestion in the stomach the process is completed in the intestines. It has little absorptive power.

The Small Intestine digests and absorbs the fats and continues the digestion of starches, sugars, fats, and proteins, when this digestion is not completed in the stomach.

The large part of the food is absorbed through the small intestine, though a small part is absorbed through the walls of the stomach and through the large intestine.

Fats are almost entirely absorbed in the small intestine. They are absorbed through the lacteals and are carried into the blood-stream.

The intestines, aside from their work of digestion and absorption, excrete bile pigment, bile salts, mucus, and other decomposition products, also such food materials as are not digested.

The Liver. The proteins, the starches (converted into maltose), and sugars pass into the liver. The sugar (including the sugar in vegetables, milk, fruits and that used for sweetening as well as the carbo-hydrates which have been changed into maltose) is converted into glycogen in the liver, stored for a time, and again broken down into a condition in which it may be absorbed into the blood.

The proteins pass through the liver but are not acted on by this organ until they again return to the liver through the blood stream, after they have been partly oxidized in the tissues. The liver further oxidizes them, putting them into condition to be excreted by the kidneys and intestines.

The liver also breaks up the worn-out red corpuscles putting them into condition to be eliminated in the bile.

It oxidizes and renders harmless poisonous substances absorbed in the food, such as fermented food products and alcohol.

The *Muscles* oxidize the fats and sugars liberating the latent heat and energy. They partly oxidize proteins which are further broken up in the liver.

The *Nerves* oxidize food materials stored in the nerve cells, providing nervous energy.

The *Lungs* absorb oxygen and throw off carbon dioxid, watery vapor, and some organic substances.

The *Kidneys* and the *Skin* excrete water, carbon dioxid, and nitrogenous waste.

The *Blood* carries the vital elements derived from the food to all the organs and tissues, keeping them alive and actively functioning. It also carries waste products to the skin, lungs, kidneys, and intestines for elimination.

FACTORS INFLUENCING DIGESTION

As before stated, it is not the food eaten, but that which the body digests and assimilates, or appropriates to its needs, which counts. Many factors influence such nourishment. The principal aids are a forceful circulation, the plentiful breathing of oxygen, and free elimination.

The
Appetite
If one has no appetite, we have been told in the past to abstain from food until the system calls for it, or to eat but a very little of the lightest food at regular meal times. This is right, but it deals with the effect and not the cause of the lack of appetite.

The chances are that this lack is due to retained waste. Whenever there is too much waste in the system, the chances are that the digestive organs will not call for more food, and when the appetite is lacking the effort should be made to see that the system is thoroughly clean.   Every muscle and tissue must be relieved of the excess of waste.   The correction of the lack of appetite, then, is not only abstinence from food, but brisk exercise, plenty of fresh air in the lungs, free drinking of water, and the elimination of the waste through the intestines, skin, lungs, and kidneys.

One should not be led into forming the habit of irregular eating, however.   The stomach forms habits and the supply of food must be regular, just as the nursing child must be fed regularly, or digestive disturbance is sure to result.

Care should be taken not to eat between meals nor to eat candy or indigestible foods.

The lack of appetite may be due to mental preoccupation which does not let the brain relax long enough for the physical needs to assert themselves. One should relax the brain in pleasant thought during the meal.

But the chief thing to bear in mind is to create the demand for food by relieving the system of its waste, by calling for more supply to the muscles through exercise, and by giving the system plenty of oxygen through deep breathing.

The appetite is partly under control of the will and may be trained.   It is more or less capricious and may be satisfied with little, or it may demand large amounts of food.   Grief or worry will destroy it, as will foul air, and overfatigue.

A voracious appetite may be due to an irritation of the nerves of the stomach or to a disturbance of digestion of one kind or another. This is shown by the fact that sometimes those with abnormal appetites are thin and undernourished because of non-digestion of the food. If the food is eaten slowly and well chewed, the desire for too great an amount will be lessened. The food will also be better digested.

The chalk-eating, clay-eating, salt-eating habits are well known. The desire is largely mental and may be treated by substituting healthful thoughts for morbid longings, and changing the monotonous or restricted diet for one more liberal.

If the appetite is lacking because of physical exhaustion, it is unwise to eat, because the digestive organs are tired, and to load a tired stomach with food, still further weakens it and results in indigestion. The better plan is to drink two glasses of cold water and lie down for an hour.

Lack of appetite and the taste for highly seasoned food may come from a monotonous diet or one that does not contain sufficient coarse food or sufficient water to stimulate peristalsis; the result is stagnation and constipation, with the disorders that follow in its train. The monotonous diet, from its effect on the mind, results in lack of desire for food. Both the condition and the appetite are often stimulated and changed by a greater variety in the kinds of food.

Care should be taken not to form the habit of using stimulants too freely, particularly with children.

Condiments and stimulants, used to make the food "appetizing," unduly stimulate the nerves, and pervert the natural taste, and foods containing their natural amount of spices or extractives no longer tempt one. Those whose nerves are highly keyed, form the habit of seasoning the food too highly.

This undue stimulation calls for more food at the time of eating than a normal appetite would demand. The taste being cultivated for the stimulant, the habit of eating too much food is formed.

A wise provision of Nature makes the system, in a normal condition, its own regulator, protesting against food when it has not assimilated or eliminated that consumed. One should learn to obey such protests and cut down the quantity when Nature calls "enough," and exercise to eliminate waste, thus creating a better assimilation. Nature does not call for more food until she has eliminated the excess of waste.

There are exceptions, however. Some phases of indigestion cause a gnawing sensation in the stomach which is often mistaken for a desire for food. This is not a normal appetite. Water will usually relieve it.

Often loss of appetite is the result of a clogging of the intestines or liver, or is due to an excess of bile, which, not having been properly discharged into the intestines, has entered the blood stream or regurgitated into the stomach. A torpid liver often expresses itself in a dull mental force, the toxins deadening the nerve cells.

The lack of desire for exercise of those living in warm climates results in a sluggish activity of the system. As a result it demands less food, and habits of excessive seasoning to stimulate the appetite have been formed.

The desire for excessive stimulants, such as salt, may be a cultivated taste and the habit should be corrected.

There is a difference between the cultivated and the normal appetite. A child rarely shows a desire for stimulants such as tea or coffee, excessive salt, pepper, pickles, catsups, etc., unless unwisely encouraged by an adult, who does it, *not because it is food for the child, but because the individual himself has cultivated a taste for it.*

It is as easy to form healthful tastes and habits of eating as unhealthful ones, and care should especially be exercised over the formation of healthful habits in the growing child.

One should not allow himself to become "finicky" or no food will give him its best service.

Time, energy, muscular activity, nerve force, and money are spent in combining, seasoning, and cooking foods in such a manner as often to render them difficult of digestion.

Let me repeat for emphasis—*when the appetite wanes, deep breathing of fresh air to supply an abundance of oxygen to oxidize the waste, thus putting it in condition to be expelled from the system, brisk exercise to accelerate the circulation, that the blood may carry the oxygen freely and that the tissues may liberate the carbon dioxid and other waste, and a copious drinking of water, are the best tonics for loss of appetite or for a lack of vitality.*

Season and Climate   The food required by the body varies according to the season of the year and the temperature. Thus, during cold weather, the body craves hot foods and drinks, and the heavier foods which furnish more heat-producing elements. In summer, the lighter foods, fruits, and the proteins supplied in green vegetables instead of in meats, are relished, and cold foods and drinks are desired as aids in equalizing the heat of the body. The total amount of food taken in summer may be lessened because so much food is not required to maintain the body heat and energy. The lessened amount puts less strain on the digestive system.

Owing to the increased perspiration, the desire for water is greater in summer, while in winter or in cool weather, from the opposite condition, the quantity of water taken is usually insufficient.

In travel, when one shifts with more or less rapidity from one temperature to another, the diet should not be altered too greatly or too suddenly; the system must be allowed time to accommodate itself to the change.

The occupation must be taken into consideration. Great muscular activity requires a more liberal diet than a sedentary habit, no matter what the climate may be.

Certain tribes that inhabit the tropics subsist almost entirely on meat, while many of the inhabitants of Russia and Norway live on breadstuffs almost to the exclusion of meat.

It is quite obvious that the food should vary according to the body needs. The **Age** needs of the adult, the child, and the infant vary. The baby may not take the food which is required by the child from the age of three to ten, and the aged, not exercising vigorously, does not need the hearty food of the growing child or the active adult. The need for food depends, however, on activity more than on years.

It is more difficult to make those in middle and old age, who are not active, realize that the body no longer needs so much food, due to the fact that it is not so actively building tissue, and that an oversupply causes a serious tax on the digestive system. It brings in its train ills which might easily be avoided by simpler habits and a little study of the actual needs of the body.

More food than the activity of the system demands, taken in later or middle life, causes most of the diseases which afflict this period. Obesity, arteriosclerosis, liver disease, gastro-intestinal diseases, biliousness, kidney diseases, gout, and allied conditions, can all be traced to an overtaxed digestive system, with faulty elimination and weakened organs. These show the rebellion of Nature at being compelled to work overtime.

While these diseases are most frequent after forty, the condition of the system which designates age is not always measured by years.

In the ordinary individual who has allowed himself to sit and become lazy in his habit of life, certain changes in the system occur and the body needs less food than is required in more active life. There are not such heavy calls on reserves for repair, either of nerve force or of material.

Unless active exercises and interests have been kept up, the muscular system begins to deteriorate, the heart action is slower, and there is a lessening of nerve tone. Relaxation of the digestive and intestinal organs occurs, peristalsis is less vigorous, and the glands become less active, owing to the lessened call for energy. From this cause, unless the amount of food is reduced in proportion to the body needs, constipation and other digestive derangements may result.

If one stops physical and mental activity at any age, the vital forces recede, muscles and vital organs become weak and inactive, and the waste of the system is not fully eliminated. Such a man at thirty or forty is physically and mentally older than the man who is in active business or is taking daily vigorous exercise, at seventy or eighty. The latter may follow the same diet which he followed at fifty, while the former should follow the diet of the old man who has stopped active work.

Young men who through excessive drafts on their vitality have exhausted their forces often act and look twice their years. For these the diet should be simple, easily digested, and nutritious, and often reduced in quantity.

Formerly it was thought that at fifty years of age a man or a woman was on the down-hill slope; they were considered " aged." Owing to the discoveries of scientific tests of the condition of arteries and vital organs, it is now known that years do not play so large a part in the matter of age.

A man or a woman at fifty, who is in vigorous mental and physical health, is in the prime of life, while many from twenty-five to thirty, who have dissipated their vital forces, may be said to have entered the age of decrepitude. The saying, " Man is as old as his arteries," should be expanded to " Man is as old as his tissues."

People have thought too long that age is a matter of years. They need to be aroused to recognize the fact that the condition of age is a matter of health of body and mind; that the spirit, which sees to it that the body which it inhabits is kept vigorous and strong by healthful and happy thoughts and an active interest in the world's affairs, is " young," no matter what the years number. Optimism and cheer keep one young; pessimism and habits of mental depression age one.

One of the encouraging signs of the times is that more and more people are learning to know that their activities need not be given up because they have reached a certain age.   If the children which formerly needed care, have grown and gone to homes of their own, the activities of the mother and father are freed to find vent in other directions.   If children no longer need immediate care, the parents have time to make better conditions for the children of others less fortunate.   They should interest themselves in public questions that affect these children and their own, indirectly if not directly.   New life and strength have been found by many by changing their activities and keeping the thoughts young and the interest vivid.   The body will respond marvelously to the mandates of the inner self.

Habit and Regularity of Eating   There is no doubt that the *habit* of eating governs one's convictions of what the system requires.   One is inclined to think that a desire for a food is a requirement of Nature; yet it may simply be the continuation of a habit due to indigestion.

Chronic abnormal functioning of the organs, such as is seen in indigestion, constipation, sluggish liver, etc., are physical habits.

If a mother feeds her babe every three hours the child will usually wake and call for food about this period.   If she has formed the habit of nursing the child every two hours, it will call for food in about two hours, even though all symptoms indicate that the child is overfed.

It is important that both child and adult establish regular and hygienic habits because the digestive juices secrete themselves at the regular periods established. *A right habit is as easily formed, and as difficult to change, as a wrong one.*

If one forms the habit of eating a certain amount of food, the stomach calls for about the same amount, and when one first begins to change the quantity it protests, whether the change be to eat more or less.

Few people form the habit of drinking sufficient water, particularly if they have been taught that water at meals is injurious. In this busy life, few remember to stop work and drink water between meals, and if not consumed at the meal time the system suffers. Many people look "dried up."

The habit of drinking two glasses of water on first arising, and six or eight more during the day is an important one.

There is no doubt that a large number of people constantly overload the digestive organs. This, as well as the bolting of food, insufficiently masticated, cannot be too strongly denounced. *All food should be chewed to a pulp before being swallowed.*

To avoid overeating, many theorists are advocating two meals a day.

Frequency of Meals

When two meals a day are eaten, the first meal should be at nine or ten o'clock in the morning and the second meal at five or six o'clock in the afternoon; whereas, for the average person who eats two meals a day, this custom means that he goes without food until the midday meal and then eats two meals within six hours, with nothing more for eighteen hours.

The argument in favor of two meals a day has been that the digestive system is inactive during sleep, and, therefore, it is not ready for a meal on arising. Pawlow's experiments, however, show that digestion continues during sleep, though less actively; and it must be borne in mind that the average evening meal is eaten about six o'clock and that there are about four waking hours between this meal and the sleep period; also, that the average individual is awake and moderately active an hour before the morning meal. This gives five waking hours between the evening and the morning meal. About the same time, five hours, elapses between the morning and the midday meal, and between the midday and the evening meal, so that three meals a day divide the digestion periods about evenly. If the amount of food supplied by two meals seems to be sufficient for the needs of the individual, and it is not practical to eat at the hours stated, then omit the midday meal.

In the strain of business life, returning at once to work, after the eating of a heavy meal in the middle of the day, calls all of the surplus blood to the brain; this, in many cases, results disastrously. For this reason, the taking of the heavy meal at night, when the system may relax and time be given to proper digestion, has come to be an institution of city life.

More frequent meals, served in lighter quantity with greater regularity, so that the system is not overloaded at any one meal, is rational for delicate or undernourished nerves and tissues.

The reason invalids or those whose digestive organs are delicate should have the heaviest meal at midday, is because the vigor of the system is greater at this time than later in the day; the increased temperature in fever in the late afternoon retards assimilation. Those whose digestive organs are delicate should not be confined to three meals a day if less food taken oftener is better borne and assimilated, but the meals should be at regular times.

Food is stored in the muscles for imme-
diate use when needed. If all of the food **Effect of**
supplied to the muscles is not used for **Exercise and Breathing**
their daily needs, an excess accumulates **on Digestion**
unless the muscles are exercised sufficiently
to use up the supply. A constant accumulation results in obesity. This condition, by overlaying the organs with fat, compresses them and hampers their activity. If the accumulation continues it ultimately causes a degeneration of the tissues. Apoplexy occurs in those carrying an excess of fat due to a weakening of the walls of the arteries of the brain.

The blood, owing to variations in the external temperature, has a tendency to retreat from the skin through contraction of the capillaries and to engorge the internal organs. Exercise brings the blood to the skin and muscles, causing the waste, broken down by the chemical activity going on every instant of life, to be picked up by the blood and carried to the elimi-nating organs. Therefore, since the blood is needed in the digestive organs during digestion, active exercise should not be taken immediately after meals.

Exercise taken in the proper amount and at proper times uses up the excess of material, benefits digestion, aids the work of the liver and intestines, keeps the circulation active, the waste eliminated, and results in a feeling of vigor and fitness for one's work whether physical or mental.

Exercise should be counted as a necessary part of one's daily activities—as necessary as eating one's meals.   If faithfully done the habit will be formed and the system will soon call for exercise as it does for food.

The young child's blood circulates freely, his breathing is unrestricted, the waste of the system is fully burned up, potential energy is released, and the result is, he must be active.   The effort of the teacher, or of those having the care of children should be, not to restrain the child but rather to direct his activity in advantageous and effective use of his energy.

A little child is an object lesson in alternating exercise, sleep, and food.   Almost every waking moment a child is squirming, twisting, and turning, using every muscle of his little body, particularly every vital organ.   No excess of waste accumulates in his tissues. The adult does not, as a rule, twist or turn or freely stretch the muscles of the vital organs.   The child and the animal stretch and yawn to start the circulation whenever they awaken from sleep.   This is instinct—Nature's law.   Man jumps out of bed and begins dressing with mind bent on the business of the day.

The necessity of oxygen is evident.   The body will subsist about forty days on the food stored within it without resupply, but it can endure only a few seconds without oxygen, because heat, occasioned by the chemical action of oxygen, is necessary to keep up the physical activity termed "life."   Carbon dioxid (carbonic acid gas) accumulates and poisons the system.

The necessity of habits of full, correct breathing cannot be too fully emphasized.

The quantity of oxygen daily consumed should equal the sum of all other food elements.[1]

Oxygen is necessary in the combustion of fats, starches, and sugars, as it is necessary in the combustion of carbon in wood or coal, and, as explained on pages 123 and 124, oxygen is necessary to keep the body warm.

Deep breathing aids digestion and assimilation, not only because of the regular exercise given to the pancreas, the spleen, the stomach, and the liver by the correct movement of the diaphragm, but also because of the latent heat which the oxygen liberates within the digestive organs and out among the tissues.

While the chemical action of food creates activity within, this activity is materially aided by exercise. Exercise and oxygen are also necessary for chemical action in tearing down waste and in putting raw material into condition to be appropriated to the body needs.

Two glasses of water in the morning and fifteen minutes of brisk exercise in well-selected movements, to start a forceful circulation and to surge the water through the digestive organs, are a daily necessity if one is to keep clean and strong within.

Exercises should be interspersed with deep breathing of *pure* air.

In breathing guard against drawing up the chest; make the muscular effort, while practicing full breathing, to expand the entire rib cage, back, front, and side.

It is as important to cleanse the body within as with-

[1] EDITOR'S NOTE:—Measurements of seventy thousand women show that sixty-two per cent. of women use only about one-half of their lung capacity and less than nine per cent. use their full capacity.

*out. It is the method employed by all men and women
who would retain strong vital forces to a ripe old age.
They fully enjoy the mere* LIVING.

Ventilation   It is of the utmost importance that one
not only forms the habit of correct, full
breathing, but also sees to it that the air in the home,
or in the place of business, is pure. A window opened
at the top and bottom is essential in any place of
business—or at least a draft through the room.

There should be plenty of *circulating* air in the
sleeping room. Many restless nights are due to
stagnant air.

Teachers find that when they keep their school-
rooms well ventilated the children are less restless, their
minds are more alert, they more quickly comprehend
what is said to them, and that both they and the
children are much less fatigued at the end of the day.

Proper ventilation, and proper exercise have so definite a bearing on the condition of the body which we
term "tired" that this subject properly follows.

**Fatigue,
Disturbed
Balance**   Since the condition of the body in fatigue
so materially affects the digestion, absorption, and assimilation of food, as well as
the elimination of waste, it is not amiss to
discuss it here.

The habit of eating when overfatigued is almost
sure to result in indigestion. Muscular or mental
activity has called the blood away from the digestive
organs and enough time has not elapsed to restore the
equilibrium.   The digestive organs are not in condition to take care of the food promptly and fermentation begins.

A few minutes of active exercise and deep breathing for the brain worker, or a half-hour of rest after muscular activity, will equalize the circulation and restore the blood to the stomach and intestines.

People fail to remember that the amount of blood in the body is a fixed quantity, and if an excess of it is called to one portion, the supply is lessened to other portions.

The regular work of the body in keeping up the heart action and the circulation requires a certain amount of energy produced by a certain amount of oxidized foodstuffs. The system in normal condition, with normal breathing, readily furnishes this energy. If more than the normal amount is used in increased work, greater combustion is necessary. The extra amount of waste which has been liberated by this extra work must also be carried away. If combustion does not take place, the extra energy is not supplied, and that required for the constant bodily needs is called on.

If the waste is not removed from the system and the energy not resupplied to the parts doing the extra work, the muscles, nerves, and tissues are then in the state termed "tired." They remain so until the circulation has carried the waste to the eliminating organs and has brought more foodstuffs to the tissues, thus restoring more energy than is needed for the work constantly going on in the body.

It must be remembered that for combustion oxygen is required and if undue energy is necessary deep breathing is imperative.

The relief, then, from the state of the body we call fatigue is in equalizing the circulation through exercise or rest, according to the occupation, and supplying oxygen through full breathing. This more forceful circulation calls the blood from the unduly distended capillaries, removes the waste, and brings a new supply of energy-building foodstuffs.

In mental work, the nerves and the brain call for the surplus energy, while in muscular work the tissues require it, hence undue work, either mental or physical, expresses itself in bodily fatigue, until the demand in all parts of the body is equalized.

When equilibrium is restored, the body is "rested."

The relief from fatigue due to mental activity is in exercise and deep breathing.

Carbon dioxid dulls the nerves of sensation and the brain action and may produce more or less stupor. It may be because the circulation in some part of the body is sluggish (most often the portal circulation through the liver), so that sufficient oxygen is not carried to that part.

Relief from this "inertness" is experienced most quickly by exercise to quicken the circulation and supply the oxygen. Exercise in one's room by the open window, or at least with the air in the room pure, is often preferable to outdoor exercise, because the body can be nude, or so loosely clothed that the oxygen may not only enter the lungs but also circulate about the skin.

Fifteen minutes of brisk exercise in one's room is better than a five-mile walk, because if the exercises are intelligently selected, every organ and tissue is used, while walking exercises only about one-fourth of the muscles.

After sleeping in a room in which the air is impure, one arises fatigued, because the supply of oxygen is insufficient to liberate the energy required for circulation and catabolism.

Harmony, either mental or physical, *is rest*.

With a little more intelligence in keeping up the supply of oxygen, in establishing correct breathing habits, and in understanding the law of distribution of circulation, which means the harmony of forces, this tired world could not only draw a deep, restful breath, but would be invigorated to enjoy life to the full.

During sleep all the processes of the body are retarded.   **Sleep**

Blood flow and breathing become slower and the digestive processes slacken. For this reason, if one goes to bed immediately after eating a heavy meal, digestion is retarded. This may react on the nerves, producing fitful or unrestful sleep. Fever or nightmare may result. The annoying, sleepy feeling which often comes on after a meal indicates a lack of balance in the system—usually that more food has been eaten than the body requires. Lessening the amount of food and increasing the exercise and the oxygen, and cleansing the intestinal tract will prevent it.

On the other hand, if the alimentary tract is entirely empty, sleep may not come because there is too much blood in the brain. A glass of hot milk or cocoa, or a couple of crackers, will call the blood to the stomach and will often aid sleep.

After eating a heavy meal, from three to three and a half hours should elapse before retiring for sleep.

The state of mind has much to do with regulating the digestive system. Cheerful thoughts keep the nerves of the entire organism in a normal state, while disagreeable thoughts cause a tense, unnatural condition.   **Influence of the Mind**

The nerves of the digestive organs are affected by the tenseness of the mind, just as are the nerves to any other part of the body. As an illustration, if one continuously thinks ugly, disagreeable thoughts, these thoughts affect the chemical activities of digestion and assimilation, resulting in an excess of acid in the blood, and actual illness results. Digestion and assimilation being impaired, the tissues become weakened, they lose their resistance, and, as a result, the organs may prolapse. We then have what is called a "vicious circle"—the mind affects the body unpleasantly and the body the mind.

We are learning to consider many factors in looking for the causes of disease, particularly those due to general weakness, or a disturbed mental state. Even the temper shown in a crying babe may affect its digestion by disturbing the normal chemical activity.

Among the blood and digestive disturbances which may result from anxiety, worry, fear, or disagreeable thoughts, are anemia, neurasthenia, indigestion, constipation, prolapsed viscera, and, in fact, all diseases which result from faulty nutrition and resultant weakened tissues.

Disagreeable thoughts affect the appetite, in fact they sometimes cause it to be entirely lost.

All so-called "new thought," "ologies," or "isms," conducive to the formation of the habit of looking on the bright side of life, or of looking for good and joy in life, of kindness, love, and helpfulness, favorably affect the digestion and consequently the health. The practice is Christian *Sense*.

The nerves control the peristaltic movements of the stomach and the action of the absorptive cells, as well as the cells which secrete the digestive juices.

Thus it is that a food which one likes is not only more palatable, but it will also digest more readily, the digestive juices flowing more freely because of the mental stimulus.

It is well, therefore, to begin the meal with something especially appetizing, that the flow of the digestive juices may be incited. For this reason, if one cares for fruit, it is an excellent custom to begin the meal with fruit, or with a well-made soup, containing protein extractives, which will stimulate the flow of digestive juices.

The habit of finishing a meal with some tasty dessert is based on the scientific principle that its palatability will cause the gastric juices to flow more freely after the meal, thus aiding in its digestion.

Dainty service in a sick-room, because of the psychic effect of a meal daintily served, is of utmost importance. Because of the effect on the mind, the sight of a meal served on soiled linen will almost stop the flow of gastric juice and will destroy the desire for food, while a meal well served on dainty linen, with garnishings and tasteful table decorations, incites the flow of gastric juices.

The careful wife and mother, who notes any failure of appetite in members of her family, should attend carefully to the garnishing of her dishes and to serving them in a neat, attractive manner; also to changing her table decorations, so far as may be consistent that the eye as well as the sense of smell and taste may be pleased and the effect of the mind on digestion be exerted.

It is strange, but it is true, that a fresh flower, or a new table decoration, may so pleasantly affect one afflicted with nervous indigestion that the meal more

readily digests, while an untidy table, or a lot of food
served untidily will retard digestion.

The custom, among hearty eaters, of serving a
plate too plentifully, destroys the appetite of one
whose digestion is not so active. Our grandmother's
overloaded table, with sufficient food of various kinds
to serve many times the number of participants,
might stimulate the appetite of hearty, strong men,
but the very sight of so much might turn the appetite
of one more delicate.

The mind must be relaxed and directed to pleasant
themes during a meal or the condition of the nerves
of the digestive organs will not permit a free secretion
of digestive juices. Chronic indigestion is sure to
result from this practice. Dinner, or the hearty meal
at night, rather than at noon, is preferable for the
business or professional man or woman, because the
cares of the day are over and the brain force relaxes.
The vital forces are not detracted from the work of
digestion.

Foods which are forced down, with a mind arrayed
against them, do not digest so readily, because the
dislike hinders the flow of the gastric juices. Any
food fails of prompt digestion when the nerves controlling the stomach are acting feebly; however,
while they digest more slowly during mental protest,
they *do* nourish the system.

Likes and dislikes are largely mental. Certain
foods continuously disagree and they should be
avoided; but many abstain from wholesome food
because it has disagreed a *few* times. It may be that
it was not the particular food but the weakness of the
stomach at the time.

Many foods disagree at certain times because of the

particular conditions regulating the secretion of digestive juices. When this condition has continued for some time it becomes chronic and a special diet is required, together with special exercises, to bring a better blood supply to stomach and intestines and to regulate the nerves controlling them, in order to correct the abnormality.

One may so form the habit of criticism or of being disgruntled or thinking he cannot eat this food and that, that his entire system suffers. Much indigestion is more mental than physical.

It can be readily seen that any tissue, playing so important a part in digestion as the blood, needs to be kept in as nearly perfect condition as possible. A vigorous circulation stimulates digestion; a poor circulation retards it. **Effect of the Circulation**

If the blood is poor in quality the digestive organs are not nourished and the digestive secretions are lessened in quantity and quality.

If the blood is imperfectly aërated it carries an insufficient supply of oxygen, combustion is lessened, and the waste, not being in a condition to be removed, remains in the tissues, stagnation results, and a slow poisoning process goes on which gradually causes the system to fail to meet the demands made on it.

The blood tissue can only be kept in condition by an adequate but not excessive amount of good food taken at the proper time, and such active exercise as will thoroughly aërate the blood by bringing the air to the smallest air cells in the lungs.

If one would fight to prevent the money used in daily exchange from being debased, he ought to be much more ready to use every means in his power to prevent a deterioration of the blood, that medium of exchange in his body on which such vital issues depend.

Tobacco and Alcohol   Tobacco and alcohol are two substances which, in excess, materially retard digestion. The effect of tobacco on the stomach is shown by its action on the small boy with his first cigar. Habituated to its use, the nerves become blunted and the nicotin narcotizes them. The use of tobacco renders the sense of taste less delicate, due to the action of the nicotin on the nerves of the taste buds. Men who use tobacco in excess miss the pleasures of taste; all food tastes much alike to them.

Tobacco, due to its action on the vagus nerve, many times causes disorders both of circulation and digestion. The starches are usually not well digested by those who are habitual users of tobacco.

Smoking before meals or when the stomach is empty often occasions nausea.

Because of its narcotic action it often exerts a soothing influence particularly in men of highly nervous temperament who are unwilling to take the necessary exercise to equalize nerve activity.

It was formerly held by physiologists that alcohol was a food, because its oxidation liberates heat, and it was assumed that this liberation of heat was the same as that freed by the combustion of fats, starches, and sugars uniting with oxygen. More recent knowledge, however, has unquestionably determined that the body decomposes alcohol into carbon dioxid and water, thus liberating heat, yet the reaction produces cold and the body requires more heat to warm it.

The blood-vessels of the skin dilate from over-stimulation, and heat is radiated faster than it is generated, so that the temperature of the body is really lowered though alcohol gives a sensation of heat. The body, therefore, loses the power to resist cold.

It was formerly used by physicians for its supposed stimulant action, but it has been determined that the apparent stimulant effect is due to irritation of the nerves, particularly of the nerves of the stomach; the temporary spur to activity is followed, however, by depression of the body forces.

The habitual use of alcohol, from overstimulation of the nervous system, affects this system, deranging it permanently, gradually lowering both mental and physical ability, and causing a catarrhal condition of the stomach and intestines.

Alcohol, therefore, even in small quantities, is a poison, and not a food.

In certain conditions it may be used in emergency to spur a flagging or failing organism to action, but owing to the facility with which the alcohol habit is acquired its use should not be continued beyond the period when its immediate action is deemed necessary.

Because tobacco and alcohol are both poisons, the healthy organism has no need of them. The diseased or deranged organism can often find greater benefit from natural remedies than from the artificial stimuli of these substances.

It is a known fact that far more men than women suffer from dyspepsia. One reason for this may be found in the prevalent habit of spitting. Smokers, in whom the irritation of the nicotin causes an excess of saliva, often suffer from gastric troubles, because they expectorate, thus wasting this valuable digestive juice.

Aside from the filthiness of the habit, which has caused laws to be enacted against it, one would think that a little reflection would cause those addicted to it to consider what it means to their health. Over-stimulation means weakened salivary glands, impaired secretion, and consequent lessened digestive power. For the sake of their own health if not from motives of decency, men should abandon the habit of expectorating.

CHAPTER VII

COOKING

THE question of the proper selection and cooking of food is so vital to the health and resultant happiness of every family, and to the strength and well being of a nation, that every one to whom cooking is entrusted should have special preparation for the work. Every girl should be given practical and thorough training in dietetics in our public schools. The study is as dignified as the study of music and art. Indeed it can be made an art in the highest conception of the term. Surely the education of every girl in the vocation in which she sooner or later may engage, either actively or by directing others, means more than education in music and drawing.

We must all eat two and three times every day; there are few things which we do so regularly and which are so vital; yet in the past we have given this subject less study than any common branch in our schools. When the dignity of the profession of dietetics is realized, the servant problem will be largely solved.

The wholesome cooking of food is as important as its selection, because the manner of cooking makes it easier or more difficult of digestion.

The necessity of a thorough education in this regard

is recognized by men who follow cooking as a profession, and a regular apprenticeship must be served before a cook is recognized as proficient. He can then command good wages.

In cooking any food, heat and moisture are necessary, the time needed varying from thirty minutes to several hours. Baked beans, and meats containing much connective tissue, as boiling and roasting cuts, require the longest time.

The purposes in the cooking of foods are:

To develop the flavor which makes the food appetizing, thus encouraging the flow of gastric juice;

To sterilize, thereby killing all parasites and microörganisms, such as the tapeworm in beef, pork, and mutton, and the trichinæ in pork;

To convert the nutrients into a more digestible form, by partially or wholly converting the connective tissue into gelatin.

According to the variety and kind, food may be roasted, broiled, boiled, stewed, baked, steamed, or fried.

Cooking of Meats		The fundamental principle to be observed in the cooking of meat concerns the retention of the juices, since these contain a large part of the nutriment. The heat develops the flavor, and the moisture together with the heat dissolves the connective tissue and makes it tender.

A choice piece of meat may be toughened and made difficult of digestion, or a tough piece may be made tender and easy to digest, by the manner of cooking.

Soups. To make meat soups, the connective tissue,

bone and muscle should be put into cold water, brought *slowly* to the boiling point, and allowed to simmer for several hours.

It must be remembered that the gelatin from this connective tissue does not contain the tissue-building elements of the albuminoids. These are retained in the meat and about the bones of the boiling piece.

The albumin of meat is largely in the blood and it is the coagulated blood which forms the scum on soup. Soup should cook slowly, or much of the nutrition is lost in the coagulated blood, or scum.

If a soup containing nutrition is desired, it must be made from boiling meat, connective tissue, and bone with marrow.

While bouillons and prepared cubes contain very little nutriment they contain the extractives, and the flavors increase the flow of digestive juices and stimulate the appetite. It is for this reason that soups are served before a meal; when they are relished, they aid a copious flow of gastric juice and saliva.

Many mistake the extractives and flavor for nourishment, thinking that soups are an easy method of taking food, but the best part of the nutriment remains in the meat or vegetables from which the soup is made, and unless one desires merely the stimulating effect, bread or crackers should supply the nourishment.

If soup meat is used in hashes the lost nutritive material in the form of gelatinoids and extractives may be restored by adding to it a cup of rich soup stock.

In preparing *Beef Tea*, the meat should be finely minced, placed in a mason jar, and a very little cold water added. It should stand an hour or two to aid in the extraction of the albumin. The jar should be then placed in a kettle of water which should be kept at the boiling point for two hours. In this way none of the nutriment is lost. Beef tea, if properly prepared and only the juice is used, is expensive, but when concentrated nourishment is necessary, cost should not figure.

The beef teas made from cubes contain the extractives and are appetizers, but they contain very little if any nutrition.

Roasting. Roasting and broiling of meats are the most universally used methods. The savage as well as civilized man prepares his meat by direct application of heat without water.

In roasting or broiling the meat is subjected suddenly to a high temperature which coagulates the albumin of the outer layers and prevents the escape of the juices. For this reason the oven should be thoroughly hot before the roast is put in. Unless the heat is sufficient to sear the surface, the moisture, or juice, will escape and the connective tissue will be toughened.

The roast should be turned as soon as one side is seared and just enough water added to prevent it from burning.

It is important to remember that the smaller the cut to be roasted, the hotter should be the fire. An intensely hot fire coagulates the exterior and prevents the drying up of the meat juice. After the surface is coagulated and seared, to prevent the evaporation of its juices, the roast should be covered so as to cook more slowly to prevent too great hardening of the surface.

Frequent basting of a roast with the fat, juice, and water in the roasting pan, still further sears the surface so that the juices do not seep through, and keeps the air in the pan moist; the heated moisture materially assists in gelatinizing the connective tissue. Roasting pans are now made which are self-basting.

Raising the temperature of the juices subjects the inner portions of the meat to moist heat and it is thus stewed in its own juices. The retention of these juices and of the extractives adds to the flavor and the palatability.

Roasted or broiled meats, if properly cooked, are more readily digested and they are usually most relished because their flavor is better retained.

Pot Roasts. For a pot roast, the meat should be well seared in fat, then a small amount of water added, and the meat cooked *slowly* at about 180 F., until done. A fireless cooker is excellent for this as for any other food needing to be slowly cooked. The juices seep out in the water and form a rich gravy which should be served with the meat.

Broiling. The same principle of quickly searing the surface applies to broiling. In broiling, however, the heat is applied direct, because the process is quicker. The meat is placed over a very hot flame or hot coals and both sides quickly seared to prevent the juice from escaping.

The object of the direct application of the heat is to enable it to quickly penetrate to the center of the chop or steak so as to coagulate the albumin and prevent the escape of the water. Meat intended for broiling should be cut at least an inch thick, as otherwise it becomes too hard and dry in the process of broiling.

Meat containing much connective tissue, such as the neck, chuck, and rump, is not adapted to broiling, because it takes too long for this tissue to become gelatinized. It may be pan broiled, a little water added, and cooked slowly until done. Prepared in this way it is cheap, nourishing, and palatable.

Steak broiled in a skillet, especially round steak which has been pounded to assist in breaking the connective tissue, is often first dipped in seasoned flour, which is well worked into it. The flour absorbs the meat juices so that none of them are lost.

When broiling meats in a skillet the skillet must be very hot before the meat is placed on it, and as soon as one surface of the meat is seared, it should be turned to sear the other side. The skillet should be kept covered so as to retain the moisture.

Boiling. One important fact, too frequently overlooked, or, perhaps, not known by many cooks, is that when water has reached the boiling point its temperature cannot be further raised by increasing the heat applied. The addition of heat only increases the production of steam and causes the water to "boil away." Therefore as soon as the water has begun to boil the gas may be turned down or the fire kept at just the level necessary to maintain the boiling. The food cooks just as soon and the fuel bills are lowered. Hard boiling has no greater effect on any food than moderate boiling.

When boiled meat is intended to be eaten—not merely boiled for soup—the water should be boiling when the meat is placed in it in order that the albumin on the surface may be immediately coagulated and prevent the escape of the nutrients into the water. It is impossible to make a rich broth and to have a juicy, highly flavored piece of boiled meat at the same time.

Meats used for boiling contain more connective tissue, therefore they require much longer cooking in order to gelatinize this tissue. They are not as rich in protein as are steaks.

Meat "shrinks" in boiling because of the escape of the water in the tissues into the water in which it is boiled. Meat may thus lose one-fourth to one-third of its weight and bulk.

Stewing. This differs from boiling in that the temperature is lower and the meat or vegetables are cut in pieces so that the water may come in contact with more of the surface thus aiding in the extraction of the juices.

The scum, which appears on the surface of a stew, is usually skimmed off and, as in the case of soups, much nutrition is lost. It should be retained, as it will disappear when the stew is thickened. It is usually removed from beef tea in order that it may not offend the eye or the capricious appetite of an invalid.

Stews should be covered and should not be cooked in too much water, as the juices are weakened and too great an amount of flour is necessary to thicken them, thus rendering them less digestible. They are cooked slowly at low temperature (130 to 160 F.) and so do not need much water.

If properly made, stews are both economical and nutritious, as no nutrition is lost in evaporation and all material save bone or gristle is utilized.

Baking. Meats, when baked, are covered with a crust, either of batter or pastry. This prevents the escape of the volatile matters, and meats thus cooked are richer, especially if they contain much fat. For this reason they are seldom suitable for invalids, or for those who have any form of stomach trouble.

Steaming. This method of cooking is applied mainly to vegetables, puddings, etc. Steamed puddings and dumplings are softer than when baked. The cover must not be removed during the time of steaming, or they may become soggy, hence less digestible.

Frying. This is the least desirable method of cooking. If a lighted match is placed near the smoke of superheated fat the fat will catch fire, showing that it is volatilizing, or being reduced to a vapor.

The extreme heat liberates fatty acids which soak into the food and render it difficult of digestion. It is wise not to employ this method of cooking unless the food is completely immersed in the hot fat by means of a wire basket. This facilitates its removal with greater ease. The surface albumin is coagulated more quickly when the food is submerged, thus preventing it from soaking up too great an amount of fat.

Deep-fat cooking requires close watching and for this reason most cooks use a skillet. Unless the skillet is very hot and the meat is turned frequently, the meat juices are lost both by evaporation and by the meat adhering to the pan.

In cooking in deep fat, if not left too long and if the fat is at the right heat, the meat fibers do not soak up the fat, because the water in the tissues is so rapidly turned to steam that the fat cannot enter; the interior thus cooks in its own juices as in roasting or broiling. Fish or chops fried in deep fat are palatable and of high flavor. Boiled fish, however, if the water is well salted to prevent too great softening, is better for invalids, as it is more easily digested.

Fish fried whole in deep fat may have the skin removed after frying. The fish fibers are thus not brought into contact with the fat. Special utensils for frying fish in this way may now be obtained.

Fats are readily absorbed in their natural condition, but, if changed by extreme heat, they are irritants.

For digestibility, therefore, boiled, broiled, and roasted foods are preferable to foods cooked in fats.

Such food as fried potatoes, mush, eggs, French toast, and griddle cakes, cooked by putting a little grease into a frying pan, are more difficult of digestion than foods cooked by any other means, particularly when the fat is heated so that it smokes.

One safe rule is to cook most foods too much rather than too little; overcooking is uncommon and harmless, while *undercooked* foods are common and difficult of digestion.

Cooking of Cereals

All partially cooked cereal foods should be cooked at least as long as specified in the directions.

One reason why breakfast foods, such as rolled oats, are partially cooked by the manufacturer, is because they keep longer.

As has been stated, the nutrients of the grain are found inside the starch-bearing and other cells, and the walls of these cells are made of crude fiber, on which the digestive juices have little effect. Unless the cell walls are broken down, the nutrients can not come under the influence of the digestive juices until the digestive organs have expended material and energy in getting at them. Crushing the grain in mills and making it still finer by thorough mastication breaks many of the cell walls, and the action of the saliva and other digestive juices also disintegrates them more or less, but the heat of cooking accomplishes the object much more thoroughly.

13

The invisible moisture in the cells expands under the action of heat, and the cell walls burst. The water added in cooking also plays an important part in softening and rupturing them. The cellulose or cell wall is also changed by heat to a more soluble form. Heat makes the starch in the cells at least partially soluble, especially when water is present.

The solubility of the protein is probably, as a rule, somewhat lessened by cooking, especially at higher temperatures. Long, slow cooking is therefore better, as it breaks down the crude fiber and changes the starch to a soluble form without materially decreasing the solubility of the protein.

The fireless cooker is particularly desirable in the cooking of cereals.

In experiments made with rolled oats at the Minnesota Experiment Station, it appeared that cooking (four hours) did not make the starch much more soluble. However, it so changed the physical structure of the grains that a given amount of digestive ferment could render much more of it soluble in a given time than when it was cooked for only half an hour.

On the basis of the results obtained, the difficulty commonly experienced in digesting imperfectly cooked oatmeal was attributed to the large amounts of glutinous material which surrounds the starch grains and prevent their disintegration. When thoroughly cooked the protecting action of the mucilaginous protein is overcome, and the compound starch granules are sufficiently disintegrated to allow the digestive juices to act. In other words the increased digestibility of the thoroughly cooked cereal is supposed to be largely due to a physical change in the carbohydrates, which renders them more susceptible to the action of digestive juices.

Pastry. Pastry is usually difficult of digestion because the fat it contains interferes with the proper solution of the starch. The objectionable features

apply to such pastry as is made by rubbing fat into
flour, as in pie crust, crust for meat pies, apple dumplings, etc. It does not apply to most puddings.
Butter or fat is used in cakes, cookies, etc., but it is
not rubbed into the flour; it is mixed with sugar and
eggs which hold it in suspension until the flour is
acted on by the liquids.

The coating of the starch granules with fat prevents
them from coming in contact with liquids. The fat
does not furnish sufficient water to enable the cells
to swell and dissolve the cell wall and so coats the
starch granules as to prevent them from absorbing
water in mixing, or saliva in mastication. This
coating of fat is not removed until late in the
process of digestion, or until the food reaches the
intestines.

The same objection applies to rich gravies, unless
the flour is dissolved in water and heated before
being mixed with the fats.

Pastry and biscuits require a somewhat hotter
temperature than bread, because the process of cooking consumes less time.

Since the root vegetables contain a
large proportion of carbohydrates, they **Cooking of Vegetables**
should be well cooked, in order that the
crude fiber may be broken and the cells fully dissolved.
Most vegetables are unpalatable and indigestible
unless, by the cooking process, the starch granules
are broken.

Vegetables are best cooked in soft water as lime
or magnesia, the chemical ingredients which make
water "hard," make the vegetables less soluble.

Vegetables and fruits become contaminated with the

eggs of numerous parasites from the fertilizers used; hence they should be thoroughly washed.

The objections to frying are as strong in regard to vegetables as to meats. The coating of fat retards digestion, as shown on page 195.

The objection to frying does not hold so strongly in the case of vegetables, such as potatoes, if fried *slowly* in fat that is not overheated, or to griddle cakes cooked slowly without smoke. It does apply, however, if the fat is sufficiently heated to smoke.

The coating of vegetables and cereals with fat prevents the necessary action of saliva on the starch globules. As previously stated, starch digestion is begun in the mouth and continued for a short time in the stomach, while the fats are not emulsified until they reach the intestine.

The starch granules in cereals and vegetables are in cells, the covering of which is composed largely of nitrogenous matter. The protein is not acted on by the saliva, and the nitrogenous matter is largely digested in the stomach. It is more easily dissolved if it is broken or softened by cooking, so that the carbohydrates can come in contact with the saliva, but if encased in fat, the gastric juices cannot digest the protein covering and the saliva cannot reach the starch until the fat is emulsified in the intestines. This means that whenever starch globules are surrounded with fat, the digestive ferments reach these globules with difficulty and foods improperly fried must be digested mostly in the intestines. For this reason, eggs, poached or boiled, are more easily digested than when fried.

Vegetables and fruits of most sorts may be baked and are usually rendered more digestible by the process.

Tubers of all sorts, if to be cooked by boiling, should be put on the fire in cold water. The gradual heating of the water allows the tuber to become warmed through before boiling begins and the interior and exterior thus are completely cooked about the same time. If placed in boiling water, the exterior, being cooked before the interior, particularly when vegetables are peeled before cooking, either separates, as in potatoes, making them "mushy," or the vegetables are served with the interior not thoroughly cooked.

Vegetables will cook as quickly and more evenly in water kept just at the boiling point as in water that is boiling hard.

All pods, seeds, or leaves, as in green vegetables, should be put in boiling water that none of the nutritive material may be lost and that the cooking action may be quickly begun.

Opinions differ markedly regarding the relative wholesomeness of raw and cooked **Cooking of Fruit** fruit. Europeans use comparatively little raw fruit, it being considered less wholesome than cooked fruit. In the United States, raw fruit is considered extremely wholesome, and is used in very large quantities; it is relished quite as much as cooked fruit, if indeed it is not preferred to it.

It has been suggested that the European prejudice against raw fruit may be an unconscious protest against unsanitary methods of marketing or handling and the recognition of cooking as a practical method of preventing the spread of disease by fruit soiled with fertilizers or with street dust. If the cooking is thorough, it insures sterilization.

As with all vegetable foods, the heat of cooking

dissolves the fiber in the cell walls. The moisture causes the cell contents to expand and rupture the walls. The change in texture occasioned by cooking renders it softer, more palatable, and more readily acted on by the digestive juices. This is obviously of more importance with the fruits like the quince, which is so hard that it is unpalatable raw, than it is with soft fruits like strawberries.

Cooking in water extracts so little of the nutritive material present in fruit that such removal of nutrition is of no practical importance unless the amount of water used is excessive. Because they contain much water fruits should be cooked in as little water as may be necessary to prevent them from burning.

The idea is quite generally held that cooking fruit changes its acid content, acid being sometimes increased and sometimes decreased by the cooking process. Kelhofer showed that when gooseberries were cooked with sugar, the acid content was not materially changed, these results being in accord with his conclusions reached in earlier studies with other fruits. The sweeter taste of the cooked product he believed to be simply due to the fact that sugar masks the flavor of the acid.

It is often noted that cooked fruits, such as plums, seem much sourer than the raw fruit, and it has been suggested that either the acid was increased or the sugar was decreased by the cooking process. This problem was studied by Sutherst, and, in his opinion, the increased acid flavor is due to the fact that cooked fruit (gooseberries, currants, plums, etc.) usually contains the skin, which is commonly rejected if the fruit is eaten raw. The skin is more acid than the simpler carbohydrates united to form a complex carbohydrate.

In some fruits, like the apple, where the jelly-yielding material must be extracted with hot water, the pectin is apparently united with cellulose as a part of the solid pulp. As shown by the investigations of Bigelow and Gore at the Bureau of Chemistry, forty per cent. of the solid material of apple pulp may be thus extracted with hot water, and consists of two carbohydrates, one of which is closely related to gum arabic. That such carbohydrates as these should yield a jelly is not surprising when we remember that they are similar to starch in their chemical nature, and, as everyone knows, starch, though insoluble in cold water, yields when cooked with hot water a large proportion of paste, which jellies on cooling.

When fruits are used for making pies, puddings, etc., the nutritive value of the dish is, of course, increased by the addition of flour, sugar, etc., and the dish as a whole may constitute a better balanced food than the fruit alone.[1]

---

[1] C. F. Langworthy, Ph.D.—In charge of Nutritive Investigations of the United States Experiment Station.

CHAPTER VIII

FOOD REQUIREMENTS OF THE SYSTEM

A S previously stated, the object of foods is:

To supply the needs of the body in building new tissue as in the growing child.

To repair tissue which the catabolic activity of the body is constantly tearing down and eliminating; and

To supply heat and energy.

The heat and energy are not alone for muscular activity in exercise or movement. It must be kept in mind also that the body is a busy workshop, or chemical laboratory, and heat and energy are needed in the constant metabolism of tearing down and rebuilding tissue and in the work of digestion and elimination.

In this chapter, a few points given in the preceding pages are repeated for emphasis.

The proteins represented in purest form in lean meat build tissue, and the carbonaceous foods, starches, sugars, and fats, supply the heat and energy.

An excess of proteins, that is, more than is needed for building and repair, is also used for heat and energy.

The waste products of the nitrogenous foods are broken down into carbon dioxid, sulphates, phosphates, and other nitrogenous compounds, and excreted through the kidneys, skin, and the bile, while the waste product of carbonaceous foods is largely carbon dioxid and is excreted mostly through the lungs.

Since the foods richest in protein are the most expensive, those who wish to keep down the cost of living, should provide, at most, no more protein than the system requires. Expensive meats may be eliminated and proteins be supplied by eggs, milk, legumes, and nuts.

The fundamental thing is to decide on the amount of protein—two to four ounces, nearly a quarter of a pound a day—and then select a dietary which shall provide this and also supply heat and energy sufficient for the day.

If the diet is to include meat, a goodly proportion of protein will be furnished in the lean meat. This will vary greatly with the different cuts of meat, as shown in Table IV, page 54. If, as often happens, one does not care for fats, then the starches and sugars must provide the heat. If much sugar is eaten less starches and fats are needed.

The normally healthy individual is more liable to take too much protein than too little, even though he abstain from meat.

If the diet is to include meat, it will be of less bulk, because the protein is more condensed; for the same reason, if it includes animal products of eggs and milk and a fair proportion of legumes, it will be less bulky than a vegetable diet. Yet unless vegetables, fruits, and plenty of water are consumed one must guard against constipation. This point is important for busy people who eat their meals in a hurry and proceed at once to active mental work.

Those who engage in physical labor are much more likely to take a complete rest for a half-hour, or an hour, after eating.   The *thinkers* seldom rest, at least after a midday meal, and those who worry seldom relax the mental force during any waking hour; their brains are as active as those of mental workers.

Every housewife, to intelligently select the daily menus for her family, needs a thorough knowledge of dietetics.   She must understand the chemistry of food that she may know food values.

The difficulty which confronts the housewife is to provide a meal suited to the needs, tastes, or idiosyncrasies of the various members of her household. Peculiarities of taste, unless these peculiarities have been intelligently acquired, may result in digestive disturbances.   As an illustration: one may cultivate a dislike for meat, milk, or eggs, as is often the case, and if the proteins for the family is largely supplied by these, the individual who omits them from the meal, eats too large a proportion of starches and sugars, and not sufficient protein—legumes, nuts, etc.   If this is long continued the blood becomes impoverished and anemia is produced.

The relief lies in *cultivating a taste* for *all foods.*

In active work, more heat is liberated, thus more fat, starches, and sugar are required for the resupply. As previously stated, if an excess of starch (glycogen) is stored in the liver, or an excess of fat in the tissues, this excess is called on to supply the heat and energy when the fats and carbohydrates daily consumed are not sufficient for the day's demands.   This is the principle in reduction of flesh.

It is interesting to note that habits of combining foods are, perhaps unconsciously, based on dietetic principles.

Meats, rich in protein, are served with potatoes or with rice, both of which are rich in starch.

Bread, containing little fat, is served with butter.

Beans, containing little fat, are cooked with pork.

Starchy foods of all kinds are served with butter or cream.

Macaroni, which is rich in starch, makes a well-balanced food when served with cheese.

Pork and beans, bread and butter, bread and milk, chicken and rice, macaroni and cheese, poached eggs on toast, and custards, form balanced foods.

A knowledge of such combinations is important when one must eat a hasty luncheon and wishes to supply the demands of the body in the least time, giving the least thought to the selection; but hasty luncheons, with the mind concentrated on other things, are to be strongly condemned.

It has been estimated that the average daily need of the adult is forty-five ounces of solid food, one-fourth animal and three-fourths vegetable. Twice as much water as solids should be taken.

The laborer, engaged in heavy muscular activity, needs and can assimilate more than the sedentary office worker. Those who work but a few hours a day require less food, as a rule, than those who work long hours.

Cold weather demands more heat-producing foods; a hot climate, inducing inactivity of body, diminishes the need for food.

The invalid needs less food than the healthy.

The inhabitant of the frigid zone needs much fat; he who lives in the tropics but little fat.

The old need less food than the growing youth or the hearty adult.

The poor must often take what he can get while the rich eat to satiety. Yet all these food needs vary with the individual and with the sex and activity.

It has been computed that the system needs daily three hundred grains of nitrogen and four thousand eight hundred grains of carbon. To obtain this amount of nitrogen if bread alone were eaten it would require four pounds of bread from the whole wheat. The carbon in this amount of bread largely exceeds that required. If eaten alone, six pounds of beef would be necessary to supply the proper amount of carbon, and twenty-three pounds of eggs. The nitrogen in this amount would far exceed the requirement.

One pint of milk, 2½ ounces of bread, and six ounces of beef are about equal in nutritive value.

One can see, therefore, why a diet composed of too great a quantity of one substance gives an overbalance of one and an underbalance of another.

Therefore, it is more economical to use some fat and sugar in the diet and less meat. More vegetables, perhaps, and more fluid should be taken by many.

Authorities vary in their estimates of the amount of food required by the individual. It varies with the activity, the season, the age, the sex, and it varies in the same individual on different days.

Billings estimates that the daily diet of a healthy, hard-working man should contain: 20 ounces (1¼ pounds) of lean meat; 22 ounces, about 1⅓ pounds or 1⅓ loaves of baker's bread; 10 ounces or about 4 medium sized potatoes; and several glasses of fluid. Since the fluid should be twice the amount of solids, this would mean about 12 glasses.

Others compute that the amount of food weighed dry, needed by the average person of sedentary habits, is as follows: For breakfast, 8 ounces; for luncheon, 6 ounces; for dinner, 9 ounces, with 48 ounces or 3 glasses of water. These two give extremes.

In active persons from 3 to 3½ ounces (about one-fourth of a pound) of nitrogenous food will replace the nitrogen lost from the body. One ounce (1 1/16 of the ordinary brick) of butter a day supplies the necessary fat, and about 15 to 20 ounces (1 to 1¼ pounds) of carbohydrate are required.

According to Thompson, from two to three pints of urine are excreted each day; ten ounces of water are lost by the lungs, and eighteen ounces are evaporated from the skin. This amount, about eighty ounces or ten glasses, must be replaced daily to maintain the body in its equilibrium of supply and demand. A part of this is supplied in the food.

These figures may be altered somewhat according to the individual or the climate as previously mentioned, but they constitute a fair average.

Dr. W. S. Hall estimates that the average man at light work requires,

each day 106.8 grams of protein[1]
57.97 grams of fat
398.84 grams of carbohydrates

These elements, in proper proportions, may be gained through many food combinations. He gives the following as an example:

Bread........................ 1 lb.
Lean Meat....................½ "
Oysters......................½ "
Cocoa........................ 1 oz.
Milk......................... 4 ozs.
Sugar........................ 1 oz.
Butter.......................½ "

[1] For table of weights see pages 357–359.

A medium-sized man at out-of-door work, fully oxidizes all waste of the system and he requires a higher protein diet—125 grams. In such event he does not require so much starch and sugar. If, on the other hand, he were to take but 106.8 grams of protein, as above, he would require more carbohydrates. One working or exercising in the fresh air breathes more deeply and oxidizes and eliminates more waste, hence he has a better appetite, which is simply the call of nature for replacing the waste.

Experiments in the quantity of food actually required for body needs, made by Prof. R. H. Chittenden, of the Sheffield Scientific School, Yale University, have established, beyond doubt, the fact that the average individual consumes very much more food than the system requires. In fact, most tables of food requirements, in books on dietetics, are heavy, yet the amount of food required as a result of Professor Chittenden's experiments would seem to be too light for a continuous diet.

Professor Chittenden especially established the fact that the average person consumes more protein than is necessary to maintain a nitrogenous balance. It was formerly held that the average daily metabolism and excretion of nitrogen through the kidneys was sixteen grams, or proportionate to about one hundred grams of protein or albuminoid food.

Professor Chittenden's tests, covering a period of six months, shows an average daily excretion of 5.86 grams of nitrogen, or a little less than one-third of that formerly accepted as necessary; 5.86 grams of nitrogen corresponds to 36.62 grams of protein or albuminoid food.

Professor Chittenden's experiments concerning the

amount of foodstuffs actually required by three groups
of men, one group of United States soldiers, a group
from the Yale College athletic team, and a group of
college professors, all showed that the men retained
full strength, with a higher degree of physical and
mental efficiency, when the body was not supplied
with more protein than was liberated by metabolic
activity, and when the quantity of carbonaceous food
was regulated to the actual requirements for body
heat and energy.

It may be well to call attention here to the fact
that most of the food elements, called on for work,
are not derived from those foods just consumed or
digested, but from those eaten a day or two previous,
which have been assimilated in the muscular tissues.

Dr. W. S. Hall gives the rations for different conditions, as shown in the following tables:

TABLE XI

RATIONS IN DIFFERENT CONDITIONS

CONDITIONS	Proteins		Fats	Carbo-hydrates		Energy in Calories
	Low	High		Low	High	
Man at light indoor work	60	100	60	390	450	2764
Man at light outdoor work	60	100	100	400	460	2940
Man at moderate outdoor work	75	125	125	450	500	3475
Man at hard outdoor work	100	150	150	500	550	4000
Man at very hard outdoor winter work	125	180	200	600	650	4592
U. S. Army rations	64	106	280	460	540	4896–5032
U. S. Navy rations	...	143	292	557	...	5545
Football team (old régime)	...	181	292	557	...	5697
College football team (new)	125	125	125	500	...	3675

TABLE XII

RATIONS VARIED FOR SEX AND AGE

VARIATIONS OF SEX AND AGE	Proteins		Fats	Carbo-hydrates		Energy in Calories
	Low	High		Low	High	
Children, two to six	36	70	40	250	325	1520–1956
Children, six to fifteen	50	75	45	325	350	1923–2123
Women with light exercise	50	80	80	300	330	2272
Women at moderate work	60	92	80	400	432	2720
Aged women	50	80	50	270	300	1870
Aged men	50	100	400	300	350	2258

The unit of measurement for the calories of energy is the amount of heat required to raise the temperature of one kilogram of water from zero to 1° centigrade or 4° Fahrenheit.

In estimating the number of calories of energy given off by the different foods, Dr. Hall represents

> 1 gram of carbohydrates as 4.0 calories
> 1 " " fats " 9.4 "
> 1 " " proteins " 4.0 "

To determine the relative energy which a food represents, it is only necessary to multiply the number of grams of protein in that food by 4, the fat by 9.4, and the carbohydrates by 4, and add the results.

Thus according to the food required for the average man at light work given on page 225:

> 106.8 grams of proteins x 4 = 427.20 calories of energy
> 57.97 " " fat x 9.4 = 544.94 " " "
> 398.84 " " carbohydrates x 4 = 1595.36 " " "

> 2567.51 = the calories of

energy required for the average man at light work.

TABLE XIII

The following gives a balanced supply for a day according to the preceding tabulation:

Amount of Food	Calories
2 tablespoonfuls fruit with sugar........	55
2 eggs...............................	140
½ pound lean meat (protein)............	243
1 pound bread........................	1206
½ pint soup	307
1 tablespoonful cocoa.................	135
2 potatoes (average size)..............	100
½ pint of milk........................	150
2 pats butter (1 cubic inch)............	119
2 tablespoonfuls sugar................	112
	2567

Dr. Chittenden's experiments would indicate that a man leading a very active life, and above the average in body weight, can maintain his body in equilibrium indefinitely with a daily intake of thirty-six to forty grams of protein, or albuminoid food, with a total fuel value of 1600 calories.

In order to bring oneself to as limited a diet as Professor Chittenden's men followed, however, it would be necessary to have all food weighed so as to be sure of the correct proportions; otherwise the actual needs would not be supplied and the body would suffer.

It is a question whether the men with whom he experimented could have followed so limited a diet for an indefinite period.

As stated, however, authorities differ on the amount of food required.

Dr. Hall suggests	106 grams of protein
Ranke suggests	100 grams of protein
Hultgren and Landergren suggest	134 grams of protein
Schmidt suggests	105 grams of protein
Forster and Moleschott suggest	130 grams of protein
Atwater suggests	125 grams of protein

A wise provision of Nature enables the body to throw off an excess of food above its needs without injury, within limitations; but, as stated, there is no doubt that the average person exceeds these limits, exhausting the digestive organs and loading the system with more than it can eliminate; the capacity for mental work becomes restricted, and the whole system suffers.

Mixed Diet versus a Vegetarian Diet From the fact that only from two to four ounces of nitrogenous food are required to rebuild daily tissue waste, it is apparent that this amount can readily be supplied from the vegetable kingdom, since nuts, legumes, and cereals are rich in proteins; yet there is a question whether a purely vegetable diet is productive of the highest physical and mental development. Natives of tropical climates live on vegetables, fruits, and nuts, and it may be purely accidental, or be due to climatic or other conditions, that these nations have not made the greatest progress. Neither have the Eskimos, who live almost entirely on meat, attained the highest development.

The greatest progress and development, both as nations and as individuals, have been made by inhabitants of temperate climates, who have lived on a mixed diet of meat, eggs, milk, grains, vegetables, fruits, and nuts. They have shown more creative force, which means reserve strength.

The Eskimo has demonstrated, however, that a diet of meat alone supplies all physical needs; the meat tissue providing growth and repair and the fat supplying all of the carbonaceous elements. The fat, as previously stated, yields more heat than starches and sugars, and Nature provides this heat for climates in which most warmth is required. This may be the reason why natives of warm climates have formed the habit of using vegetables and grains for their heat and energy rather than meat. It is also the natural reason why man in temperate climates eats more meat in winter than in summer.

An unperverted, natural instinct will always be found to have a sound physiological basis. For example, if, by reason of some digestive disturbance, one has become emaciated, all of the fat having been consumed, and the cause of the disturbance is removed by an operation or otherwise, one is seized with an almost insatiable desire for fat, often eating large chunks of the fat of meat or large quantities of butter or cream at a meal. When obstructions are removed, Nature makes immediate effort to readjust her forces.

Those who object to eating meat should study carefully to learn if the proper proportion of protein is supplied with each day's rations. The legumes— peas, beans, nuts, and grains—must be supplied. While the wheat kernel contains twelve per cent. of protein, the white flour does not contain as large a percentage and it will be noted by reference to Tables II and III, that the majority of fruits and vegetables contain little nitrogenous substance.

Unless the whole of the grain and the legumes form a goodly proportion of the diet the danger is in consuming too large a bulk of waste and too much starch in a purely vegetable diet.

In a vegetarian diet, one is liable to eat too freely of cereals; as a result, the liver becomes clogged and torpid and the stomach and intestines are deranged and rendered incapable of full digestion and absorption.   The clogged system refuses to assimilate more food.

It follows, therefore, that, unless one is a thorough student of dietetics, the mixed diet is by far the safest to follow.

One can better run short of starch or fat in one day's rations than to be short of protein, because if the two or four ounces daily requirement is not provided the tissues are consumed and the blood is impoverished.   It is a rare condition in which a reserve of glycogen and fat is not stored in the system.   On the other hand, an excess of nitrogenous foods calls for a very active circulation and plenty of oxygen in the system.

It has been held that the vegetarian has a clearer brain, and, if this be true, it may be due to the fact that he is not eating too much and thus his system is not overloaded.

Experience, however, does not prove that he has greater mental, physical, and moral power and efficiency.

In fasting, likewise, the mental power is at first clear and forceful, but the reason becomes unbalanced if the fast be too prolonged.

A complete diet may be selected without animal flesh, but including animal products of eggs, milk, cream, and butter, together with vegetables, fruits, cereals, and nuts, yet, if the vegetable diet be selected, the legumes, the

*whole of the grains, and nuts, must be given their share
in each day's rations.*

Each year sees an increase in the number
of travelers. The question of diet many
times is of great importance. For those of
abundant means the question is simplified, oftentimes,
by the railway dining-car service, but for those who
from economic reasons must patronize the wayside
railway restaurants or other eating places, the diet
question is not so easily solved.

Diet when Traveling

A carefully planned lunch-box is often an aid to
the preservation of regular habits and a preventative
of digestive disturbances, due to a sudden and radical
change of diet.

The inactivity and sedentary habit enforced by a
long journey, in which there is small chance for exercise, generally causes constipation. The shaking of
the boat or train also aids this, as it interrupts normal
peristalsis. The motion of the boat or train often
produces nausea and vomiting and thus deranges the
digestive organs.

Greasy or illy prepared food hastily eaten at a
lunch counter provokes various gastric and intestinal
ills.

The danger of infected or polluted water complicates
the problem, especially when the sick or infants are
involved. Many an attack of typhoid fever has
been traced to the drinking water used during a
vacation trip.

The invention of the vacuum bottle has solved one
need of the traveler. The invention of the electric
heater has solved another.

Sterilized and cooled milk may be carried by means

of the vacuum bottle for use with children or the sick, and the portable stove will enable the boiling and sterilizing of water, when a larger supply is needed than can be carried in a vacuum bottle.   By its means, also, a hot drink can be prepared for the aged, the invalid, or other individual, when necessary, as in an emergency.

All fried and greasy food and unripe fruits should be avoided.

One had better lessen the amount of food than suffer the gastric difficulties occasioned by too much fatty food.

Hard whole wheat crackers with fruit and milk can be had at almost any eating house.   These give a well-balanced meal and are often preferable to prepared dishes.   Fresh fruit, especially the acid fruits, should form a large part of the diet.

The traveler, on extended journeys, should always provide some of the easily carried condensed foods, so that if the food obtained by the way is unpalatable or illy prepared, or in case food is unobtainable, the needs of the system may be met.   Beef meal, whole wheat or oatmeal crackers, malted milk, chocolate, meat extracts, etc., occupy little space and may often prove invaluable.

Tablets of soda and also of lime are easily carried and may be used when soda water or lime water is needed as in nausea or indigestion.

If it is possible, the water drunk while traveling should be boiled.

The bowels must be kept active and fresh fruits and water are the best aids in accomplishing this.

The remedies recommended for car sickness or sea-sickness are legion; what is an aid in one case is almost or quite without avail in another.   Lemon juice or a slice of lemon in the mouth is generally of most avail, though lime water in some cases has proven of service.   Attacks can often be mitigated or avoided by not starting on a journey when overtired, by light eating for several days previous to beginning a journey, with care in securing good elimination and plenty of fresh air.

If traveling by boat a reclining chair on deck is far preferable to lying in a berth in a stuffy stateroom.

Nausea can often be prevented or remedied by deep breathing or by the sipping of hot water with a little soda.

CHAPTER IX

DIETS

*B*EFORE *giving any diets, let me first of all impress
the importance of eating slowly, of good cheer, of
light conversation during a meal, and of thoroughly
masticating the food. Remember it is the food assimilated which nourishes.*

The following diets allow sufficient food for average conditions, when the vital organs are normal.

Fruit, as previously stated, contains a very small
quantity of nutrition. It is more valuable for its
diuretic effect, and to stimulate the appetite; for this
reason it may well be eaten before a meal.

The citrus fruits tend to neutralize too high acidity
of the blood, increasing its alkalinity. For this reason,
also, they are best before a meal, particularly before
breakfast; they have a more laxative and cleansing
effect if eaten before the other food. The custom
has been, however, to eat fruits after dinner for dessert
and they are so given in the following menus.

Table XI (page 207) gives the total amount of protein, carbohydrate, and fat needed daily for the work
of the body. The method of determining the number
of calories produced by each variety of food is also
given on page 208.

By a little study of the food one ordinarily eats in

connection with this tabulation and the tables given on pages 233 to 241, it can be determined whether the food taken each day is well or illy balanced and whether one is eating too much or not enough.

Table XIII (page 209) gives the balanced supply for a day of the most commonly used foods and may be consulted as a basis from which to work in constructing balanced meals.

[Because of the wide variation in methods of preparing food in the home, an exact and absolute standard cannot be fixed.

All foods contain combinations of mineral salts, particularly calcium (lime), sodium, magnesium, and potassium. In each food, however, some mineral predominates. For instance, potatoes contain both calcium and potassium but the potassium content is larger than the calcium. For this reason when potassium salts are needed in a diet, potatoes and other potassium-containing foods make a valuable contribution. When potassium needs to be limited these foods should be omitted from the diet. When calcium is needed, as in growing children, calcium-containing foods should be made a large part of the diet.

In conditions of health the construction of a balanced diet is a comparatively simple matter. In conditions of disease, however, the question of diet is often one that can only be solved by a skilled dietitian, after a chemical analysis. Unfortunately, the number of these in the United States is not large and their services are not available in many cases in which they are needed.

A diet in which the acid-forming elements are in excess will ultimately result in a lessening of the alkalinity of the blood. The blood then, to maintain its balance, withdraws alkaline substances from the tissues. A balance must, therefore, be maintained between the acid and alkaline foods. This has a bearing on scurvy and also in gout.

Foods which are called acid, that is, they tend to lessen the normal alkalinity of the blood, are, oats, barley, beef, wheat, eggs, rice, and maize. When the proportion of acid in the blood is too great the supply of these foods should be lessened.

Alkaline foods, or those which leave no acid residue, are carrots, turnips, potatoes, onions, milk, blood, peas, lemon and orange juice, and beans. These may be used when there is too much acid in the system.

Neutral foods are sugar, the vegetable oils, and animal fats.

All the content of the foods must be taken into consideration in building a diet, the carbohydrate, fat, and protein being considered as well as the mineral. A consideration of the mineral content, however, should not be neglected. One-eighth grain of iron is taken daily in the ordinary mixed diet. The fact that in one quart of milk, according to Hutchinson, there are ½ grains of calcium shows how valuable this food is to the growing child for bone and tissue building. It must also be considered when constipation results from a milk diet. Milk and its derivatives are poor in iron, while meat, fish, potatoes, fruits, and bread are poor in calcium. Animal foods are rich in sodium; vegetables and fruits in potassium.

The following shows the foods which contain mineral salts, in larger proportions.

Calcium (lime)	Milk contains 1½ grams of lime (calcium) in every quart; next in lime content come eggs, then cereals, especially rice, radishes, asparagus, spinach, veal, olives (16%), apples and strawberries. Tea, coffee, rhubarb, and cabbage cause deposits of the oxalate of calcium.
Potassium Sodium Magnesium	Egg yolk, potatoes, apples, lemons, limes, oranges, olives (60%) and strawberries.
Sulphur	Cabbage, asparagus, fibrin of meat, eggs, casein of milk, corn, turnips, cauliflower, and asparagus.
Iron	Yolk of egg, beef, spinach, dandelions, apples, lettuce, lentils, strawberries, navy beans, peas, potatoes, wheat, and oatmeal.
Phosphorus	Meat and most vegetables.

A knowledge of the carbohydrate content of foods is useful also in making up a diet, especially in diabetes. Friedenwald and Ruhrah give the following in their order:

Less than 5%	String beans, asparagus, spinach, pickles, lettuce, cucumbers, greens, celery, Brussels sprouts, rhubarb, sauerkraut, tomatoes, ripe olives, cauliflower.
From 5 to 10%	Leeks, eggplant, pumpkin, kohlrabi, cabbage, radishes, collards, watermelon, mushrooms, beets, okra, strawberries, turnips, lemons, rutabagas, squash, musk melons, peaches, onions, cranberries.
From 10 to 15%	Blackberries, green onions, oranges, green olives, tomato catsup, currants, raspberries, apricots, parsnips, pears, apples, lima beans.

From 15 to 20%   Nectarines, huckleberries, cherries, green peas, almonds, potatoes, succotash, fresh figs, prunes, grapes, baked beans, green corn.

Over 20 %   Plums, boiled potatoes, bananas, sweet potatoes.

In the following menus the effort has been to give a correct balance of the various food elements with the approximate calories furnished by each meal. They are suggestive only and may be varied according to the season of the year, the habits of work, or the tastes of the individual, care being taken to preserve the relative proportions.

For instance, if much starch or fat is taken at a meal and little protein, the balance should swing in the other direction for another meal, the amount of protein being increased and that of carbohydrate decreased.

Common sense must rule in the matter, as one individual would be illy fed on a diet which would be entirely adequate for another of more sedentary habit and weaker digestion. All the habits of life such as exercise, breathing, and mental activity must be taken into consideration.

As previously remarked, there must be a variety in the diet which will stimulate the appetite, and, unless the tastes of the various members of a family are capricious, they may be gratified.

If potatoes are not relished rice may be substituted.

Plain bread may be varied by rolls or biscuits.

Well-masticated nuts may supply the protein usually served in meat and are often a welcome change.

The protein balance is important as this substance

is the basis for growth and repair of the tissues of the body.

When the protein balance of the family meal is provided by meat, if for any reason one member of the family does not care for meat, the protein may be supplied by eggs, or by the legumes as shown on pages 232–234.

Let me repeat that everyone should watch his likes and dislikes in the matter of food and guard against allowing himself to become finicky; he should not cultivate a dislike for a food which may disagree with him at a certain time or the taste of which he does not like, if that food is wholesome.

Remember that the likes and dislikes for food are largely matters of cultivation and one misses much enjoyment and much of health which comes from a well-nourished body by habitually sitting down to a table in a pessimistic frame of mind because the food served does not suit the fancy.

It is very difficult for a mother to provide a meal which suits each member of her family and consideration for her as well as for self should teach one to guard against a critical attitude.

The following is an example of a badly balanced menu. It was given a family, including a child, by a mother who "had no time to study foods. She gave her folks what was the easiest to get and filled them up the quickest." This mother may have wasted hours in gossip with the neighbors, or on "fancy work."

Breakfast

Rolls with butter
2 cups coffee

Luncheon
Fried sweet potato
Bread and butter
Prunes
Tea

Dinner
Macaroni with cheese
Bread and butter
Boiled potato
Boiled rice with milk
Tea with milk and sugar

The cardinal sin of such a diet is in the lack of protein, the great predominance of starch, and the inadequate supply of fat. An excessive amount of sugar, however, was taken in the tea. This was taken to satisfy the taste, not realizing that the system demanded it for energy.

The child was given one egg and one slice of bread for breakfast. Being a light eater it asked for no more, but her mother wondered why the child was so pale and suffered from constipation.

No water was given with any meal.

There are thousands of such illy nourished children in our schools, lacking in brain power and readily subject to infection, because of badly combined or poorly prepared food.

The number of calories in such a diet may suffice to sustain life, but the balance is insufficient, the amount inadequate, the tissues are not repaired, the secretions lack some of their necessary ingredients or are scanty, and the functions of the body are not well performed.

Sedentary Occupation
The following diet is for one who has attained full growth and who exercises no more than to walk a few blocks a day.

The diet may seem light, but when one is sitting indoor most of the time, and has little outdoor exercise, less waste protein is oxidized and less starch, fat, and sugar are required for heat and energy. If too much carbonaceous food is consumed, one will store up too much and become too large. If more protein is consumed than is oxidized and eliminated one is liable to various derangements of the system.

Every person at sedentary employment should exercise each day without fail, being particular to bring a thorough circulation to the vital organs. He should fully inflate his lungs many times a day and see to it that the air in the room is pure.

In nearly all of the following menus coffee and tea have been omitted because, as before stated, they are not foods but *stimulants*, and the caffein and thein may overstimulate the nerves and the heart. They sometimes retard digestion. Some other warm drink should be substituted when there is digestive disturbance, or when the digestion is weak. They should never at any time be used strong. They are used simply for their pleasing flavor, or for warmth.

The following diet is suggested for one of sedentary habit who is not exercising and does not use up much mental or physical energy.

DIET I

Breakfast

Fruit
Cereal coffee or toast coffee
Dry toast (one slice), or one muffin, or one gem
1 slice of crisp bacon
1 egg

If one has taken brisk exercise, or is to take a brisk walk of two or three miles, a dish of oatmeal or some other cereal, with cream and sugar, may be added.

Luncheon

Fruit

Creamed soup or purée

Meat, cheese or peanut butter sandwich, or two thin slices of bread and butter

Cup of custard, or one piece of cake, or two cookies

If purée of peas or beans is used the sandwich may be omitted and one slice of bread is sufficient. If the soup contains much cream or is made of corn or potato, the cake or cookies may be omitted.

Dinner

Meat, gravy, potatoes or rice

One vegetable (green peas, green beans, cauliflower, greens, corn. Do not use dried baked beans or dried peas with lean meat)

Salad or fruit

Ice cream or pudding, such as bread, rice, tapioca, cornstarch, or chocolate, or an easily digested dessert.

Diet II gives the calories of energy required by a business man or brain worker who uses much mental force.

DIET II

Breakfast

1	orange without sugar	100
1	shredded wheat biscuit with sugar and cream	175
2	slices bacon	75
2	tablespoonfuls creamed potato	160
1	egg	70
2	slices toast with butter	250
1	baked apple	85
2	cups cocoa	80
		995

Luncheon

1	bowl oyster stew	250
6	crackers	120
		370

Dinner

½	pint clear soup with croutons	75
1	portion beefsteak	433
2	tablespoonfuls green beans	70
2	baked potatoes (medium size)	90
2	slices bread	175
1	pat butter	33
2	tablespoonfuls rice pudding with raisins and cream	450
		1326
		995
		370
		2691

Diet III gives approximately the calories required for one taking moderate exercise.

DIET III

Breakfast

	Fruit with sugar	100
2	tablespoonfuls oatmeal with cream and sugar	170
1	piece broiled fish four inches square	205
2	slices buttered toast	250
1	cup coffee with cream and sugar	125
		850

Luncheon

2	tablespoonfuls beans baked with bacon	150
1	baked apple with cream	200
1	cup cocoa	68
2	slices bread (thin) with butter	200
		618

Dinner

½ pint purée (vegetable)	150
1 portion boiled mutton	300
2 potatoes (medium size)	90
2 slices bread and butter	250
2 tablespoonfuls scalloped tomato	150
2 tablespoonfuls brown betty or peach tapioca with light cream	300
1 cup coffee with cream and sugar	125
	1365
	850
	618
	2833

For the Girl or Boy from 13 to 21 There is no time in life when one needs to be so watchful of the diet as during these years. Growth is very rapid and much protein is needed to build tissue, particularly to build the red blood corpuscles. Anemia may be produced by a faulty diet or by one which lacks eggs, meat, fresh vegetables or fruit, particularly in developing girls.

The red meats, the yolk of eggs, spinach and all kinds of greens are important articles of diet at this time, because of the iron which they contain. They should be supplied freely. Butter and milk are valuable and *regular exercises with deep breathing are imperative.*

If the appetite wanes, be sure that the girl or boy is getting sufficient brisk exercise in the fresh air.

DIET IV

Breakfast

Fruit
Oatmeal, shredded wheat biscuit or triscuit, or some other well cooked cereal with cream and sugar

One egg, boiled or poached (cooked soft), or chipped beef in cream gravy

Cereal coffee, toast coffee, or hot water with cream and sugar

Buttered toast, gems, or muffins

Luncheon

Cream soup, bean soup, or purée with crackers or dry toast

Bread and butter

Fruit and cake, or rice pudding, or bread, tapioca, cocoanut, or cereal pudding of any kind, or a cup of custard, or a dish of ice cream

Dinner

Meat (preferably red meat)

Potatoes

Vegetables, preferably spinach, or greens of some kind, or beets boiled with the tops

Graham bread

Fruit, graham bread toasted or graham wafers. Cake of some simple variety.

Candy (small quantity)

A growing child is usually hungry when it returns from school, and it is well to give a little easily digested food regularly at this time, but not sufficient to destroy the appetite for the evening meal. Irregular eating between meals, however, should be discouraged. An egg lemonade is easily digested and satisfying. If active and exercising freely, craving for sweets should be gratified to a limited extent.

The growing boy or girl takes from six to eight glasses of water a day.

Overeating, however, should be guarded against for many of the dietary habits of adult life are formed in this period, and the foundation of many dietetic difficulties and disturbances of the system are laid.

If one is not hungry at meal time, the chances are that he is not exercising sufficiently in the fresh air.

Thorough mastication should be insisted on.

One should encourage the habit of eating hard crusts or hard crackers to exercise the teeth and to insure the swallowing of sufficient saliva.

The schoolboy or schoolgirl, anxious to be out at play, is especially liable to bolt the food or to eat an insufficient amount. This should be especially guarded against and parents should insist on the proper time being spent at meals.

The dislike for meat or for certain vegetables or articles of food, which develops in this period, should be guarded against. All wholesome food should be made a part of the diet and the child should not be indulged in its likes or dislikes, but should be instructed in overcoming these.

Very few foods disagree at all times with a normal child and if they do the cause usually lies in a disordered digestion which needs to be restored by more careful attention to exercise, deep breathing, and to elimination of the waste of the system.

The Athlete   The young man active in athletics needs practically the same food as given in Diet IV, yet more in quantity. He needs to drink water before his training and at rest periods during the game.

If he is too fat, he should train off the superfluous amount by exercise and by judiciously abstaining from much sugars, starches, and fats.

Diets for reduction, however, must be governed by the condition of the kidneys and the digestive organs.

Deep breathing habits are imperative though he must be careful not to overtax lungs or heart by hard continuous straining, either at breathing or at exercise.

The man engaged in muscular work requires plenty of food; he can digest **The Labor-ing Man** foods which the professional or business man, or the man of sedentary habits, cannot.   He will probably be able to drink coffee and tea without any disturbance to nerves or to digestion.   In his muscular work he liberates the waste freely and needs fats, starches, and sugars to supply the heat and energy. This is especially true of men who work in the fresh air; the muscular action liberates waste and heat and the full breathing freely oxidizes the waste, putting it in condition to be excreted through lungs, skin, kidneys, and intestines.

He should have more meat, eggs, and nitrogenous foods, and he also needs more carbonaceous foods to supply heat and energy, as given in Diet V.   Three hearty meals a day are necessary.

His muscular movements keep the circulation force-ful and the vital organs strong so that his diet may be almost as heavy as that of the football player. Meat or eggs, twice a day, with tea or coffee, and even *pie* may be eaten with impunity.   He needs a good nourishing breakfast of bacon and eggs or meat, also potatoes, or a liberal allowance of bread and butter, corn bread, muffins, etc.

DIET V

Breakfast

		Calories
4	tablespoonfuls fresh or stewed fruit with sugar	100
3	tablespoonfuls oatmeal with milk and sugar	200
1	portion ham four inches square with fat	200
2	eggs	140
2	cups coffee with cream and sugar	250
2	slices bread and butter	250
		1140

Luncheon

2	sandwiches (cheese)	300
1 ·	sandwich (marmalade)	125
1	pint of milk	200
1	slice cake or pie	100
		725

Dinner

½	pint oyster stew or vegetable purée	100
2	baked potatoes	100
4	tablespoonfuls macaroni with tomatoes and butter sauce	200
4	slices thick bread and butter	500
2	portions roast beef (fat)	400
2	cups coffee	250
1	slice pie	100
		1650
		1140
		725
		3515

Condition of Age　　　The following constitutes an average which will supply the daily requirement for the aged, or for one at any age whose organs are not functioning strongly.

DIET VI

Breakfast

Cereal, well cooked, with cream or sugar.   Oatmeal is preferable
  because it is laxative
One egg, boiled, poached, or baked (soft)
One slice of toast
Cereal coffee

Dinner

Bouillon or soup
Meat—small portion
Potato (preferably baked)
One vegetable
Cup custard, or bread, rice, or other light pudding with lemon
  cream sauce

Supper

Soup
Bread and butter
Stewed fruit
Tea

These individuals need little meat.   Tea, if used,
should not be strong and, for reasons given on page
104, should never be allowed to steep.

If the habit of life is active, if one exercises regularly,
and if the constitution is vigorous and the body not
too encumbered with fat, a greater variety and amount
of food may be allowed, but great regularity should
be observed concerning the diet and the hours for
meals.   Thorough mastication is more than ever a
necessity.

If inclined to constipation, or if the kidneys are
inactive, grapes or an apple, or some fruit, well
chewed, may be eaten just before retiring.

Careful attention must be given to securing thorough
removal of waste by attention to the eliminative
organs, not overloading them.

TABLES OF USE IN MAKING UP BALANCED DIETS

The following table from Dudley Roberts is of material help in making up combinations of foodstuffs for balanced diets:

FOOD STUFF	Quantity		Calories of Energy	Grams of Protein
Milk	8 oz.	1 glass	160	8.4
Skim milk	8 oz.	1 glass	80	8.0
Cream	8 gm.	1 tsp.	20	0.2
Condensed milk (sweetened)	20 gm.	hp. tsp.	50	1.8
Condensed milk (unsweetened)	20 "	" "	40	2.0
Chocolate powd.	10 "	" "	90	1.2
Beef juice, beef tea, bouillon, clear soup	5 oz.	teacup	5-30	1.3
Cream soup	8 "	soup plate	100-250	
Sugar	10 gm.	hp. tsp.	40	
Egg (whole)	50 "	1	70	
Egg (yolk)	—	1	55	2.4
Butter	10 gm.	1 in. cube	65	0.6
Cheese	" "	" "	45	3.0
Meat and fish (lean)	50 "	hp. tbsp.	60	12.0
Meat (medium fat)	" "	" "	100	7.0
" (very fat)	" "	" "	150	4.0
Oysters (small)	8 "	1	3	0.5
Oysters (large)	25 "	1	10	1.5
Crackers	3-10 "	1	12-30	3-6
Cereals (cooked)	30-40 "	teacup	110-150	3-5
Cereals (prepared)	5-7 "	hp. tsp.	18-25	0.5-0.7
Shredded wheat	30 "	1	100	3.0
Triscuit	15 "	1	50	1.5
Peas(fresh or canned)	35 "	hp. tbsp.	25	2.0
Peas (dried)	25 "	" "	100	6.0
Beans (dried)	25 "	" "	90	5.0
Beans (fresh or canned)	30 "	" "	30	1.0
Potatoes (medium size)	90 "	1, 3 in.long	80	1.0
Jelly (sweet)	—	teacup	50-100	—
Apples	100 "	1	40	0.2
Oranges	125 "	1 med. size	60	0.5
Bananas	50 "	1 med. size	45	0.7
Dried fruit (prunes, etc.)	100 "	1 saucer medium	100-200	1-3

The following tables[1] are exceptionally valuable in compiling diets in various combinations. One can readily determine the number of grams in various servings of different foods. For example: a small serving of beef (round), containing some fat, weighs 36 grams; 40 per cent., 14.4 grams, is protein, and 60 per cent., 21.6 grams, is fat (no carbohydrates). One ordinary thick slice of white, home-made bread weighs 38 grams; 13 per cent., 4.94 grams, is protein; 6 per cent., 2.28 grams, is fat, and 81 per cent., 30.78 grams, is carbohydrate.

The proportion of proteins, carbohydrates, and fats required by the average individual as suggested on page 208 can be readily made up from various combinations of foods. Each individual may ascertain whether he is taking too much food, or too large a proportion of proteins or of carbohydrates or fats.

TABLE OF 100 FOOD UNITS

NAME OF FOOD	"Portion" Containing 100 Food Units (approx.)	Wt. of 100 Calories		Per cent. of		
		Grams	Oz.	Proteid	Fat	Carbo-hydrate
COOKED MEATS						
†Beef, r'nd, boiled (fat) ...Small serving...		36	1.3	40	60	00
†Beef, r'd, boiled (lean)....Large serving...		62	2.2	90	10	00
†Beef, r'd, boiled (med.) ..Small serving...		44	1.6	60	40	00
†Beef, 5th rib, roasted....Half serving....		18.5	0.65	12	88	00
†Beef, 5th rib, roasted....Very small s'v'g.		25	0.88	18	82	00
‡Beef, ribs boiled........Small serving...		30	1.1	27	73	00
*Calves foot jelly.....................		112	4.	19	00	81

[1] These are from *Food and Dietetics* (Norton), published by the American School of Home Economics, Chicago. They are used in a number of schools of Domestic Science and in the Dietetic kitchens in hospitals.

NAME OF FOOD	" Portion " Containing 100 Food Units (approx.)	Wt. of 100 Calories		Per cent. of		
		Grams	Oz.	Proteid	Fat	Carbohydrate

COOKED MEATS—*Continued*

*Chicken, canned........One thin slice...		27	0.96	23	77	00
*Lamb chops, broiled, av..One small chop..		27	0.96	24	76	00
*Lamb leg, roasted.......Ord. serving....		50	1.8	40	60	00
†Mutton, leg, boiled.....Large serving...		34	1.2	35	65	00
†Pork, ham, boiled (fat).Small serving...		20.5	0.73	14	86	00
†Pork, ham, boiled.......Ord. serving....		32.5	1.1	28	72	00
†Pork, ham, r'st'd (fat)...Small Serving...		27	0.96	19	81	00
†Pork, ham, r'st'd (lean)..Small serving...		34	1.2	33	67	00
†Veal, leg, boiled........Large serving...		67.5	2.4	73	27	00

VEGETABLES

*Artichokes, av. canned................		430	15.	14	0	86
*Asparagus, av. canned.................		540	19.	33	5	62
*Asparagus, av. cooked................		206	7.19	18	63	19
*Beans, baked, canned....Small side dish..		75	2.66	21	18	61
*Beans, Lima, canned....Large side dish..		126	4.44	21	4	75
*Beans, string, cooked....Five servings....		480	16.66	15	48	37
*Beets, edible portion, cooked............Three servings..		245	8.7	2	23	75
*Cabbage, edible portion...............		310	11	20	8	72
Carrots, cooked........Two servings...		164	5.81	10	34	56
*Cauliflower, as purchased.............		312	11.	23	15	62
*Celery, edible portion.................		540	19.	24	5	71
Corn, sweet, cooked.....One side dish...		99	3.5	13	10	77
*Cucumbers, edible pt..................		565	20.	18	10	72
*Eggplant, edible pt...................		350	12.	17	10	73
Lentils, cooked......................		89	3.15	27	1	72
*Lettuce, edible pt....................		505	18.	25	14	61
*Mushrooms, as purchased.............		215	7.6	31	8	61
Onions, fresh, edible pt..............		200	7.1	13	5	82
*Onions, cooked........2 large s'v'gs...		240	8.4	12	40	48
Parsnips, cooked....................		163	5.84	10	34	56
*Peas, green, canned.....Two servings...		178	6.3	25	3	72
*Peas, green, cooked......One serving....		85	3.	23	27	50
Potatoes, baked........One good sized..		86	3.05	11	1	88
*Potatoes, boiled........One large sized..		102	3.62	11	1	88
*Potatoes mashed(creamed)One serving....		89	3.14	10	25	65
*Potatoes, chips........One-half s'v'g...		17	0.6	4	63	33
*Potatoes, sweet, cooked..Half av. potato..		49	1.7	6	9	85
*Pumpkins, edible pt..................		380	13.	15	4	81
Radishes, as purchased...............		480	17.	18	3	79
Rhubarb, edible pt...................		430	15.	10	27	63
*Spinach, cooked.......Two ord. s'v'gs..		174	6.1	15	66	19
Squash, edible pt....................		210	7.4	12	10	78
*Succotash, canned.......Ord. serving...		100	3.5	15	9	67
*Tomatoes, fresh as purchased............Four av........		430	15.	15	16	69
Tomatoes, canned....................		431	15.2	21	7	72
*Turnips, edible pt.......2 large s'v'gs....		246	8.7	13	4	83
Vegetable oysters....................		273	9.62	10	51	39

NAME OF FOOD	"Portion" Containing 100 Food Units (approx.)	Wt. of 100 Calories		Per cent. of		
		Grams	Oz.	Proteid	Fat	Carbo-hydrate
FRUITS (DRIED)						
*Apples, as purchased..................		34	1.2	3	7	90
Apricots, as purchased.................		35	1.24	7	3	90
*Dates, edible portion....Three large.....		28	0.99	2	7	91
*Dates, as purchased....................		31	1.1	2	7	91
*Figs, edible portion......One large.......		31	1.1	5	0	95
*Prunes, edible portion...Three large.....		32	1.14	3	0	97
*Prunes, as purchased..................		38	1.35	3	0	97
*Raisins, edible portion.................		28	1.	3	9	88
*Raisins, as purchased..................		31	1.1	3	9	88
FRUITS (FRESH OR COOKED)						
*Apples, as purchased....Two apples.....		206	7.3	3	7	90
Apples, baked.........................		94	3.3	2	5	93
Apples, sauce...........Ord. serving....		111	3.9	2	5	93
Apricots, cooked.......Large serving...		131	4.61	6	0	94
*Bananas, edible pt.......One large.......		100	3.5	5	5	90
*Blackberries...........................		170	5.9	9	16	75
Blueberries...........................		128	4.6	3	8	89
*Blueberries, canned...................		165	5.8	4	9	87
Cantaloupe............Half ord. serv'g..		243	8.6	6	0	94
*Cherries, edible portion................		124	4.4	5	10	85
*Cranberries, as purchased..............		210	7.5	3	12	85
*Grapes, as purchased, av...............		136	4.8	5	15	80
Grape fruit...........................		215	7.57	7	4	89
Grape juice............Small glass.....		120	4.2	0	0	100
Gooseberries..........................		261	9.2	5	0	95
Lemons...............................		215	7.57	9	14	77
*Lemon juice...........................		246	8.77	0	0	100
Nectarines...........................		147	5.18	4	0	96
Olives, ripe.............About seven....		37	1.31	2	91	7
Oranges, as purchased, av.One very large..		270	9.4	6	3	91
*Oranges, juice..........Large glass.....		188	6.62	0	0	100
Peaches, as purchased, av.Three ordinary..		290	10.	7	2	91
*Peaches, sauce.... .....Ord. serving....		136	4.78	4	2	94
Peaches, juice..........Ordinary glass...		136	4.80	0	0	100
Pears..................One large pear..		173	5.40	4	7	89
*Pears, sauce..........................		113	3.98	3	4	93
Pineapples, edible p't'n, av..............		226	8.	4	6	90
*Raspberries, black.....................		146	5.18	10	14	76
Raspberries, red.......................		178	6.29	8	0	92
Strawberries, av.......Two servings....		260	9.1	10	15	75
*Watermelon, av........................		760	27.	6	6	88
DAIRY PRODUCTS						
*Butter................Ordinary pat....		12.5	0.44	0.5	99.5	00
*Buttermilk.............1½ glass		275	9.7	34	12	54
*Cheese, Am., pale.......1½ cubic in.....		22	0.77	25	73	2
*Cheese, cottage.......4 cubic in.......		89	3.12	76	8	16
*Cheese, full cream.......1½ cubic in.....		23	0.82	25	73	2
*Cheese, Neufchatel......1½ cubic in.....		29.5	1.05	22	76	2
*Cheese, Swiss..........1½ cubic in.....		23	0.8	25	74	1

NAME OF FOOD	"Portion" Containing 100 Food Units (approx.)	Wt. of 100 Calories		Per cent. of		
		Grams	Oz.	Proteid	Fat	Carbo-hydrate

DAIRY PRODUCTS—*Continued*

NAME OF FOOD	"Portion"	Grams	Oz.	Proteid	Fat	Carbo-hydrate
*Cheese, pineapple.......1½ cubic in.....		20	0.72	25	73	2
*Cream.................¼ ord. glass		49	1.7	5	86	9
Kumyss............................		188	6.7	21	37	42
*Milk, condensed, sweet'nd		30	1.06	10	23	67
*Milk, condensed, unsw't'nd..............		59	2.05	24	50	26
*Milk, skimmed.........1½ glass		255	9.4	37	7	56
*Milk, whole............Small glass.....		140	4.9	19	52	29
Milk, human, 2d week.................		162	5.7	11	47	42
Milk, human, 3d month................		171	6	7	46	47
*Whey.................Two glasses.....		360	13	15	10	75

CAKES, PASTRY, PUDDINGS, AND DESSERTS

NAME OF FOOD	"Portion"	Grams	Oz.	Proteid	Fat	Carbo-hydrate
*Cake, chocolate layer ....Half ord. sq. pc.		28	0.98	7	22	71
*Cake, gingerbread.......Half ord. sq. pc..		27	0.96	6	23	71
Cake, sponge...........Small piece.....		25	0.89	7	25	68
Custard, caramel......................		71	2.51	19	10	71
Custard, milk...........Ordinary cup...		122	4.29	26	56	18
Custard, tapioca........Two-thirds ord..		69.5	2.45	9	12	79
*Doughnuts ....Half a doughnut		23	0.8	6	45	49
*Lady fingers............Two..........		27	0.95	10	12	78
*Macaroons.............Four...........		23	0.82	6	33	61
*Pie, apple ....One-third piece..		38	1.3	5	32	63
*Pie, cream ....One-fourth pc ..		30	1.1	5	32	63
*Pie, custard ....One-third piece..		55	1.9	9	32	59
*Pie, lemon ....One-third piece..		38	1.35	6	36	58
*Pie, mince ....One-fourth piece		35	1.2	8	38	54
*Pie, squash ....One-third piece..		55	1.9	10	42	48
Pudding, apple sago		81	3.02	6	3	91
Pudding, brown betty...Half ord. s'v'g...		56.6	2.	7	12	81
Pudding, cream rice.....Very small s'v'g.		75	2.65	8	13	79
Pudding, Indian meal....Half ord. s'v'g...		56.6	2.	12	25	63
Pudding, apple tapioca...Small serving ...		79	2.8	1	1	98
Tapioca, cooked........Ord. serving....		108	3.85	1	1	98

SWEETS AND PICKLES

NAME OF FOOD	"Portion"	Grams	Oz.	Proteid	Fat	Carbo-hydrate
*Catsup, tomato, av		170	6.	10	3	87
Candy, plain...........................		26	0.9	0	0	100
Candy, chocolate......................		30	1.1	1	4	95
*Honey ....Four teasp'ns...		30	1.05	1	0	99
*Marmalade (orange)....................		28.3	1	0.5	2.5	97
Molasses, cane.....................		35	1.2	0.5	0	99.5
*Olives,green,edible,portion Five to seven ..		32	1.1	1	84	15
*Olives, ripe, edible portion Five to seven...		38	1.3	2	91	7
*Pickles, mixed........................		415	14.6	18	15	67
*Sugar, granulated.......Three heap'g t sp. or 1½ lumps...		24	0.86	0	0	100
*Sugar, maple..........Four teaspoons..		29	1.03	0	0	100
*Syrup, maple..........Four teaspoons..		35	1.2	0	0	100

NAME OF FOOD	" Portion " Containing 100 Food Units (approx.)	Wt. of 100 Calories		Per cent. of		
		Grams	Oz.	Proteid	Fat	Carbo-hydrate

NUTS, EDIBLE PORTION

*Almonds, av...........Eight to 15.....		15	0.53	13	77	10
*Beechnuts.............................		14.8	0.52	13	79	8
*Brazil nuts............Three ord. size..		14	0.49	10	86	4
*Butternuts...........................		14	0.50	16	82	2
*Cocoanuts............................		16	0.57	4	77	19
*Chestnuts, fresh, av..................		40	1.4	10	20	70
*Filberts, av.............Ten nuts.......		14	0.48	9	84	7
*Hickory nuts..........................		13	0.47	9	85	6
*Peanuts, av............Thirteen double.		18	0.62	20	63	17
*Pecans, polished........About eight.....		13	0.46	6	87	7
*Pine nuts (pignolias).....About eighty....		16	0.56	22	74	4
*Walnuts, California.....About six.......		14	0.48	10	83	7

CEREALS

*Bread, brown, average...Ord. thick slice..		43	1.5	9	7	84
*Bread, corn (johnny cake) av.....................Small square..		38	1.3	12	16	72
*Bread, white, home made Ord. thick slice..		38	1.3	13	6	81
*Cookies, sugar.........Two...........		24	0.83	7	22	71
Corn flakes, toasted......Ord. serving....		27	0.97	11	1	88
*Corn meal, granular, av..2½ level tbsp...		27	0.96	10	5	85
Corn meal, unbolted, av..Three tbsp......		26	0.92	9	11	80
*Crackers, graham.......Two crackers...		23	0.82	9.5	20.5	70
*Crackers, oatmeal.......Two crackers...		23	0.81	11	24	65
*Crackers, soda..........3½ "Uneedas"..		24	0.83	9.4	20	70.6
*Hominy, cooked.......Large serving...		120	4.2	11	2	87
*Macaroni, av....................		27	0.96	15	2	83
Macaroni, cooked.......Ord. serving....		110	3.85	14	15	71
*Oatmeal, boiled.........1½ serving.....		159	5.6	18	7	75
*Popcorn.............................		24	0.86	11	11	78
*Rice, uncooked.......................		28	0.98	9	1	90
*Rice, boiled...........Ord. cereal dish .		87	3.1	10	1	89
*Rice, flakes............Ord.cereal dish..		27	0.94	8	1	91
*Rolls, Vienna, av......One large roll....		35	1.2	12	7	81
*Shredded wheat........One biscuit.....		27	0.94	13	4.5	82.5
*Spaghetti, average....................		28	0.97	12	1	87
*Wafers, vanilla.........Four...........		24	0.84	8	13	71
Wheat,flour,e't'e w'h't,av.Four tbsp......		27	0.96	15	5	80
*Wheat, flour, graham, av.4½ tbsp.......		27	0.96	15	5	80
*Wheat, flour, patent, family and straight grade spring wheat, av.......Four tbsp......		27	0.97	12	3	85
*Zwiebach..............Size of thick slice of bread......		23	0.81	9	21	70

MISCELLANEOUS

*Eggs, hen's, boiled......One large egg...		59	2.1	32	68	00
*Eggs, hen's, whites......Of six eggs......		181	6.4	100	0	00
*Eggs, hen's, yolks.......Two yolks......		27	0.94	17	83	00
*Omelet.............................		94	3.3	34	60	6

NAME OF FOOD	"Portion" Containing 100 Food Units (approx.)	Wt. of 100 Calories		Per cent of		
		Grams	Oz.	Proteid	Fat	Carbo-hydrate

MISCELLANEOUS—*Continued*

NAME OF FOOD		Grams	Oz.	Proteid	Fat	Carbo-hydrate
*Soup, beef, av........................		380	13.	69	14	17
*Soup, bean, av.........Very large plate.		150	5.4	20	20	60
*Soup, cream of celery ....Two plates.....		180	6.3	16	47	37
*Consommé.............................		830	29.	85	00	15
*Clam chowder.........Two plates.....		230	8.25	17	18	65
*Chocolate, bitter........Half-a-square...		16	0.56	8	72	20
*Cocoa................................		20	0.69	17	53	30
Ice cream (Phila.).......Half serving....		45	1.6	5	57	38
Ice cream (New York) ...Half serving....		48	1.7	7	47	46

* *Chemical Composition of American Food Materials*, Atwater and Bryant, U. S. Department of Agriculture, Bull. 28.

† *Experiments on Losses in Cooking Meats* (1900–03), Grindley, U. S. Department of Agriculture, Bull. 141.

‡ Laboratory number of specimen, as per *Experiments on Losses in Cooking Meats.*

TABLES SHOWING AVERAGE HEIGHT, WEIGHT, SKIN SURFACE, AND FOOD UNITS REQUIRED DAILY WITH VERY LIGHT EXERCISE

Boys

Age	Height in Inches	Weight in Pounds	Surface in Square Feet	Calories or Food Units
5	41.57	41.09	7.9	816.2
6	43.75	45.17	8.3	855.9
7	45.74	49.07	8.8	912.4
8	47.76	53.92	9.4	981.1
9	49.69	59.23	9.9	1043.7
10	51.58	65.30	10.5	1117.5
11	53.33	70.18	11.0	1178.2
12	55.11	76.92	11.6	1254.8
13	57.21	84.85	12.4	1352.6
14	59.88	94.91	13.4	1471.3

Diets

GIRLS

Age	Height in Inches	Weight in Pounds	Surface in Square Feet	Calories or Food Units
5	41.29	39.66	7.7	784.5
6	43.35	43.28	8.1	831.9
7	45.52	47.46	8.5	881.7
8	47.58	52.04	9.2	957.1
9	49.37	57.07	9.7	1018.5
10	51.34	62.35	10.2	1081.0
11	53.42	68.84	10.7	1148.5
12	55.88	78.31	11.8	1276.8

MEN

Height in Inches	Weight in Pounds	Surface in Square Feet	Proteids	Calories or Fats	Food Units Carbo-hydrates	Total
61	131	15.92	197	591	1182	1970
62	133	16.06	200	600	1200	2000
63	136	16.27	204	612	1224	2040
64	140	16.55	210	630	1260	2100
65	143	16.76	215	645	1290	2150
66	147	17.06	221	663	1326	2210
67	152	17.40	228	684	1368	2280
68	157	17.76	236	708	1416	2360
69	162	18.12	243	729	1458	2430
70	167	18.48	251	753	1506	2510
71	173	18.91	260	780	1560	2600
72	179	19.34	269	807	1614	2690
73	185	19.89	278	834	1668	2780
74	192	20.33	288	864	1728	2880
75	200	20.88	300	900	1800	3000

WOMEN

Height in Inches	Weight in Pounds	Surface in Square Feet	Proteids	Calories or Fats	Food Units Carbo-hydrates	Total
59	119	14.82	179	537	1074	1790
60	122	15.03	183	549	1098	1830
61	124	15.29	186	558	1116	1860

WOMEN—*Continued*

Height in Inches	Weights in Pounds	Surface in Square Feet	Proteids	Calories of Fats	Food Units Carbo-hydrates	Total
62	127	15.50	191	573	1146	1910
63	131	15.92	197	591	1182	1970
64	134	16.13	201	603	1206	2010
65	139	16.48	209	627	1254	2090
66	143	16.76	215	645	1290	2150
67	147	17.06	221	663	1326	2210
68	151	17.34	227	681	1362	2270
69	155	17.64	232	696	1392	2320
70	159	17.92	239	717	1434	2390

NOTE.—With active exercise an increase of about 20 per cent. total food units may be needed.

DIETARY CALCULATION WITH FOOD VALUES IN CALORIES PER OUNCE

Breakfast	Proteids	Fats	Carbo-hydrates	Total
Gluten gruel, 5 oz.	23.5	1.0	30.0	
Soft-boiled egg	26.3	41.9		
Malt honey, 1 oz.			86.2	
Creamed potatoes, 5 oz.	15.0	40.0	104.0	
Zwiebach, 2 oz.	22.8	52.8	171.6	
Pecans, ¾ oz.	8.4	141.0	13.4	
Apple, 5 oz.	2.5	6.5	83.0	
	98.5	283.2	488.2	869.9

DIETARY CALCULATION WITH FOOD SERVED IN 100 CALORIES PORTIONS

Dinner	Portions in serving	Proteids	Fats	Carbo-hydrates	Total
French soup	½	10	20	20	
Nut sauce	1	29	55	16	

Dinner—Continued	Portions in serving	Proteids	Fats	Carbo-hydrates	Total
Macaroni, egg	1	15	59	26	
Baked potato	2	22	2	176	
Cream gravy	½	5	33	12	
Biscuit	1½	20	2	128	
Butter	1	1	99		
Honey	2			200	
Celery	¼	4		21	
Apple juice	½			50	
	10¼	106	270	649	1025

HOURLY OUTGO IN HEAT AND ENERGY FROM THE HUMAN BODY
AS DETERMINED IN THE RESPIRATION CALORIMETER
BY THE U. S. DEPT. OF AGRICULTURE

Average (154 lbs.)	*Calories*
Man at rest (asleep)............................	65
Sitting up (awake).............................	100
Light exercise..................................	170
Moderate exercise..............................	190
Severe exercise.................................	450
Very severe exercise.....	600

16

CHAPTER X

IN the dietetic treatment of any disordered organ, the object must be to give that organ as much rest from its regular work as is consistent with keeping up the general nutrition of the system. The stomach and intestines and liver are so closely allied that, when one is affected, the others are liable to affection also, and the dietetic treatment is regulated accordingly.

In abnormal conditions it is necessary to say that the food must be regulated according to the case. Yet, broadly speaking, a diet largely of protein, which is digested in the stomach, rests the intestines and stimulates the liver, and a diet largely of carbohydrates rests the stomach, because the gastric juice is not active in starch digestion.

When the body is not in normal condition, because certain elements are lacking in the blood, these elements must be supplied in larger proportions in the food, and the case is one for a food chemist, or for one who has made food conditions a study.

The better medical colleges, recognizing the importance of proper food in health and disease, have in the last few years broadened their curriculum to include the subject of dietetics. Educated physical culturists and food specialists, for the correction of deranged conditions of the system, due to poor circulation and abnormal nerve and blood conditions, are doing much of the corrective work, due to the fact that instruction has not been given in the medical colleges.

Diets for the reduction of an abnormal amount of fat must also be governed according to the individual condition.

In the early stages of various diseases, when toxins are being produced, as a rule the system is not properly eliminating the waste, and it is often advisable to abstain from food for from one to three days, according to conditions. Brisk exercise, deep breathing, and a free use of water are desirable. A laxative is often recommended.

The diets given here for abnormal conditions are to enable those in charge of an invalid to gain an intelligent understanding of the needs of the system and to supply those needs through the proper foods. In serious cases, however, special diets will be ordered by the medical attendant to suit the needs of the individual.

A chemical analysis of the blood and the excretions is often the only method of determining just the diet in the individual case.

Government chemical laboratories in charge of efficient chemists should be so located as to be accessible to every physician.

The system readily excretes an excess of vegetable products, and, as a rule, no acute difficulties result from such an excess. Such chronic difficulties as constipation, torpid liver, and indigestion, however, frequently result when an excess of starch is taken above that consumed in energy.

On account of the readiness with which putrefaction occurs in protein products, care should be taken not to consume these in too great proportion.

A study of the physical ailments of thousands of women has shown, by the constituents in the blood and the condition of the different organs of the digestive system, the habitual taste for foods. One can usually determine which food the individual has formed a habit of eating, because the system will show a lack of the elements which that patient has denied herself on account of her likes and dislikes.

It is necessary to change the mental attitude toward certain foods before the system will readily assimilate them; thus, as stated, *a taste for foods which the body requires should be cultivated.*

Every mother, with growing children, should be a thorough student of the chemistry of food. If the child's bones do not increase sufficiently in size and strength after the second year, care in the selection of foods rich in protein and phosphates of lime and magnesium may correct it. Such a child should have scraped meat and whole wheat bread with milk and eggs.

If the child stores up too much fat, increase the amount of exercise and of oxygen consumed, and either cut down the proportion of sweets and starches or decrease the quantity of food and require more thorough mastication.

If one is thin and undernourished, chemical analysis of the contents of the stomach, intestines, and urine is sometimes desirable. The nerves should be relaxed, and proper food, exercise, and breathing should accompany medical treatment, if medicine is needed. Often an entire change in thought and diet are helpful.

Sometimes a torpid condition of the liver and sluggish activity of the intestines are indicated.   Special
exercises to stimulate this activity and to encourage
correct poise and deep breathing are most essential.
The mind must often be stimulated and an interest
be awakened, directing the thoughts in new channels.

Worry and tensity of thought are among the chief
causes in the majority of cases of lack of flesh and of
a very large number of blood and digestive disorders.

In anemia there is either a decrease in   **Anemia**
the number of red blood corpuscles or an
insufficient amount of blood.   When there are too
few red blood corpuscles, "oxygen carriers," the necessary quantity of oxygen is not furnished the tissues
and the system becomes clogged with waste.   The
patient easily tires and is disinclined to exercise, thus
the decreased number of red corpuscles are not kept
in forceful circulation and the carbon dioxid is not
freely thrown off by the lungs; this further aggravates
the condition.

Since the blood is made from the foods assimilated,
the point is to supply food which builds blood tissue.
Exercise and deep breathing will encourage the elimination of waste and promote a forceful circulation
which insures nourishment to the tissues.   As stated,
it is the food assimilated, not always the amount
eaten, that counts.

In this condition it is of vital importance that one
keep up a good circulation; the stomach, intestines,
liver, and spleen must be strengthened through exercise and deep breathing of pure air, for the red blood
corpuscles are oxygen carriers, and the insufficient
supply must do double duty or the waste of the system

will not be oxidized and eliminated, and the blood-forming organs will further fail in their task.

Exercise must be graded to the case, being gentle at first so as not to overtire the easily fatigued muscular system. It should be intelligently directed to the joints and to the vital organs, particularly to the liver and intestines, that they may be kept in normal activity. The exercises must be followed with plenty of rest, and accompanied by deep breathing. The habit of full breathing is one of the most effective agencies in correction of anemia, because the red blood corpuscles must carry their full quota of oxygen or the system is clogged with waste. Oxygen also rejuvenates these corpuscles.

Unless the blood furnished to the tissues is of good quality and contains sufficient oxygen, the nutrition of the body suffers, the activity of the various organs is hindered, and the health becomes impaired. Functional derangements, particularly in the digestive tract follow, and faulty digestion and difficult absorption further impoverish the blood.

The work, therefore, in the correction of anemia, lies in foods which build blood and in daily exercise and deep breathing of fresh air, accompanied by rest.

The windows at night should admit a good circulation of air through the sleeping room, and as much time as possible should be spent in the open air.

Anemia occurs many times in growing girls, due to an improperly balanced diet, caused by a capricious appetite and by the habit of satisfying this appetite with sweets, pickles, etc.

The body, during growth, needs increased nutritive material, not only to replace the waste, but also to meet the demands for new building material for the various organs, particularly the brain and the nervous system. Overwork either in school or in industrial occupations, the hasty eating of meals, or insufficient amounts of food, also aid in reducing both the quantity and quality of the blood.

Worry is one chief cause of anemia.

Insufficient sleep, due to late hours, further increases the tension of the nerves and lowers the vitality, causing depression which interferes with digestion.

When the red blood corpuscles are decreased the oxidation of the fats is interfered with, because oxygen is necessary to burn the fat. The non-use of the fatty material causes it to be stored in the tissues so that the body often appears well nourished and plump. The muscles, however, are flabby and weak and usually the pallor of the skin shows the lack of coloring matter in the blood.

The digestive organs are often weak. They must not be overloaded or the very object of the extra feeding will be defeated. In such cases the food must be taken in less quantity and more frequently. Also a diet rich in albumin and iron must be supplied.

It will often be found that one whose blood is lacking in hemoglobin and in the proper proportion of red blood corpuscles has had a dislike for the foods rich in iron, or perhaps through poverty, or some other cause, has not been able to get the right kind of food.

The yolks of eggs, the red meats (such as steak, mutton, or the breast of wild game) and the deeply colored greens (such as spinach, chard, dandelions, etc.) contain a goodly proportion of iron. The dark leaves of lettuce, celery, and cabbage contain iron;

these vegetables are apt to be bleached before being marketed.

It is better, in anemia, to take the yolks of two eggs than one whole egg, as the iron is in the yolk. A good way to take the yolks of eggs is in egg lemonade or in eggnog, with a little flavoring.

Anemia sufferers have usually formed the habit of eating starches and sweets. It will usually be found that they have no desire for vegetables containing iron, or for meats rich in albuminoids, and this habit is shown in the blood composition. They often eat the white of the egg and discard the yolk, rich in iron. Tact and persuasion will often be necessary to induce them to take the proper foods.

If constipation is present, whole wheat bread, oatmeal, stewed prunes, grapes, stewed or baked apples, and oranges, should be taken freely.

When the anemic individual is thin, he should take as much fat food as the system will assimilate. Bacon is well digested and palatable. Fat may be taken in milk, cream, and butter.

The food must be made attractive to tempt the appetite, which is usually poor, and within reason one should be allowed any wholesome food which he desires. Condiments often stimulate the stomach and intestines to better action.

Vinegars, because of their action on the blood, should not be allowed nor rich pastries and sauces.

Beef may be scraped and made into sandwiches or used in purées and meat broth, which may also have a beaten egg in it.

The following is a suggestive diet in anemic conditions:

DIET VII

One pint of milk, to be sipped slowly before arising.

Breakfast

Fruit
Broiled steak or two eggs, soft-boiled, poached, or baked, with
    bacon
Cereal coffee, chocolate, or cocoa
Toast, or graham, or whole wheat bread, or graham or corn
    muffins; butter

Middle of the Forenoon

Lemonade with a tablespoonful of beef juice (not beef extract)
    or with a beaten egg, or a
Glass of egg malted milk, or an
Eggnog

Lunch

Split pea or bean soup with toast and butter, or scraped beef
    sandwich with lettuce
Fruit or vegetable and nut salad (no vinegar)
Fruit, fresh or stewed
Bread with plenty of butter
Cake
A glass of milk, cocoa, or chocolate—preferably milk

Middle of Afternoon

Egg lemonade or eggnog of two eggs beaten in boiling milk with
    sugar and spices

Dinner

Bouillon
Tenderloin steak, roast beef, or lamb chops
Baked potato
Spinach, beet, or dandelion greens
Custard, fruit gelatin, or cornstarch pudding, or rice with lemon
    cream or butter sauce
Bread and plenty of butter
Glass of milk or weak tea

When appetite is persistently absent, attention should be paid to the eliminative organs in order to remove all clogging of the system by retained waste.

If the stomach and intestines are prolapsed as a result of improper nourishment and resultant weak tissues, rest in bed, with special exercises which will replace the organs and strengthen the supporting tissues, is required.

STOMACH DISORDERS

Most chronic cases are due to worry; to improper hygiene, such as irregular meals; fat and greasy foods; hasty eating; too much sweets; insufficient mastication, with resulting lack of saliva; wrong choice of foods; too frequent eating, giving the stomach no rest; too large an amount of food; too highly spiced foods; coffee or tea; a general run-down condition, with a weakness of muscles of the stomach, due to insufficient blood supply; to a weakened or over-strained condition of nerves controlling the stomach; and usually to insufficient exercise and fresh air.

Indigestion or Dyspepsia Indigestion or dyspepsia is the broad term commonly applied to most chronic stomach and intestinal difficulties, due, not alone to structural disease or to displacements, but also to their inability to perform their normal functions. The term includes troubles arising from so many different causes that in each case the cause must be determined and remedied before definite results can be attained through diet.

The most usual is that the gastric glands are pouring out an insufficient amount of secretion; almost always there is a deficiency of hydrochloric acid. In some cases in which the food has irritated and inflamed the stomach there may be a sufficient secretion of this acid, but an inflamed stomach throws off more mucus and the extra quantity of mucus neutralizes the hydrochloric acid.

When the acid is deficient or absent, the proteins are not well digested and the food may ferment; bacteria may produce putrefactive changes and the formation of gas. The gas interferes with the movement of the diaphragm, pressing it against the heart, causing pain and even palpitation.

Indigestion is usually accompanied by constipation, or by irregular action of the intestines.

Plenty of fresh air, and exercise, directed definitely to muscles and nerves of the stomach, that it may be strengthened by a better blood supply, as well as exercises and deep breathing to build up the general health, should be systematically followed.

Easily digested food, well masticated, and regular meals served daintily, will gradually regulate digestion.

Food should not be of too great a variety at one meal. It must be simple and well prepared; when nerves and muscles are weak it should be served less in quantity but more frequently. Sometimes light food every hour or every two hours is best.

Cheerful constructive thoughts are the very best of medicine for digestive derangements.

A glass of cold water from one-half to an hour before the meal will cleanse the stomach by washing out the mucus and will promote the secretion of saliva and the gastric juices.

The intelligent medical treatment of stomach

difficulties is aided by a chemical analysis of the stomach contents. If the stomach is not secreting normal proportions of pepsin or hydrochloric acid, the deficiency of either can be determined. Such chemical analysis will alone determine what elements are lacking.

Permanent relief must lie in gaining a good circulation of blood through the entire body and through the stomach, that it may be strengthened and thus enabled to secrete these elements in proper proportions.

Nervous Indigestion This is due to the general depleted condition of the nerves. In such cases the entire nervous system should be regulated through exercise, breathing, rest, and a change of thought. Physicians usually recommend change of scene to cause a change of thought.

The diet should be light and laxative, and low in protein. Cream soup, bread and milk, malted milk, buttermilk, cream, fruits, crackers and milk, custards, egg lemonade, and gruels, furnish easily digested food.

Tea, coffee, much meat, fried food, highly spiced food, pastry, candies, pickles, alcohol, and tobacco should be avoided.

When the walls of the stomach are weak and distended or prolapsed, light food served in small quantities at regular but more frequent periods is preferable to a hearty meal, which further distends the stomach walls. The stomach does not secrete sufficient gastric juices to digest a meal large enough to supply the needs of the system, if food is taken only three times a day.

When a loss of weight occurs, it usually indicates a failure to *assimilate* rather than the failure to eat a sufficient amount of food. A good circulation, particularly through the vital organs, must be established; deep full breathing of fresh air, and regular and complete rest periods, should be observed.

Usually, in chronic cases, a dietitian, or a physician, is not called until the condition has prevailed for so long that other complications have set in and the patient has lost much flesh. It takes months to pull the system down and it takes months of following of proper hygiene to build it up.

This involves an inflammation of the mucous lining of the stomach and is a most common phase of indigestion. In acute cases the physician is called at once. He can then treat the case in its initial stage and cause a much more rapid recovery.

Gastritis or Catarrh of the Stomach

Acute Gastritis is accompanied by nausea and vomiting and the patient should refrain from taking food for at least two days. To allay thirst a tablespoonful of water may be held in the mouth for a few moments without swallowing it. A slice of lemon may be sucked if water excites vomiting, or cold carbonated or acidulated waters may be sipped, a teaspoonful at a time, every ten or fifteen minutes. Rest of both body and mind must be obtained.

After two days begin the nourishment with water and a small portion of liquid food (not over two ounces) every two hours. Toast tea, made by pouring hot water over toast, oatmeal, or barley gruel (thoroughly strained so that no coarse matter may irritate the stomach), limewater and milk, and egg lemonade are easily digested. Increase the quantity on the fourth day and lengthen the time between feedings to three hours. Gradually increase the diet, adding semiliquid food, noted on pages 237–238, soft-boiled eggs, moistened toast, raw oysters, etc., slowly returning to the regular bill of fare.

Avoid any food difficult of digestion and any vegetable containing coarse fiber.   Care in the diet must be observed for several weeks or a relapse may occur.

Chronic Gastritis is accompanied by a thickening of the mucous lining of the stomach. It is usually caused by prolonged use of irritating foods and the regulation of the diet is of utmost importance. Alcohol is a common cause. The difficulty begins gradually and the relief will be gradual.

There is an excessive secretion of thick, tenacious mucus which prevents the gastric juices from mixing with the food. The resulting fermentation of food causes heartburn and produces much gas. Thirst may be excessive.

The stomach needs washing. The washing may be accomplished by drinking two glasses of hot water at least an hour before breakfast, followed by stomach exercises, to cause a surging of the water through the stomach. This may be followed by a glass of cold water.

This may be uncomfortable at first, causing a full feeling, and one may begin by drinking one glass, followed by stomach exercises, gradually taking another glass within a half-hour of the first. This, by means of the exercises, will wash out the mucus.

A glass of cold water half an hour before each meal is recommended here, as well as for relief of indigestion.

In many cases as much as a pint of slimy mucus collects in the stomach during the night. When the stomach cleansing by means of water drinking is impossible, the physician often uses a stomach tube.

Chronic gastritis, in any of its phases, is frequently accompanied by constipation, which reacts on the stomach, and the diet should be as laxative as possible, without irritating the lining of the stomach.

In case an acute attack occurs, which is likely in chronic cases, the diet under "Acute Gastritis" should be followed.

Pancreatinized milk is an excellent food in both chronic and acute cases especially when they are severe. This is prepared by putting "pancreatin" a pancreatic ferment (trypsin) into fresh milk. Preparations of "pancreatin" are sold in the drug stores. Pepsin may be used in the same way for making peptonized milk.

The pancreatinized milk does not form hard curds and readily passes through the stomach for digestion in the intestine. The taste is rather bitter; it may be disguised by flavoring. This may be given for a few days, followed by milk and lime water, barley and toast water, kumys, oatmeal gruel, meat juices, scraped meat (raw, boiled, or roasted), broths thickened with thoroughly cooked cereals, ice cream, egg lemonade, gelatins and whipped cream, custards and raw oysters.

Fruit in the morning and just before retiring aid the intestines. Two prunes chopped up with one fig, or a bunch of grapes, or an apple, just before retiring may be eaten to assist the action of the intestines and the kidneys.

Almost all fruits contain acids which increase the peristalsis, and the resultant flow of gastric juice. Cooked pears, stewed or baked apples, prunes, and dates are mild fruits which may be used if they agree. The juice of an orange on arising may be used if relished.

All cereals should be thoroughly cooked.

The white meat of chicken, well masticated, is readily digested.

After an acute attack, as the solid food is resumed, it should be given regularly and in small amounts.

Thorough mastication is important. The food should be chewed until it is reduced to a pulp.

Fats and food cooked in fat must be avoided. Dried beef, lean boiled ham, and salt fish agree better with some than fresh meats. All sweets must be forbidden. Starchy foods are apt to produce "sour stomach."

Avoid meat with tough fiber, too fat meat (pork), sausage, lobster, salmon, chicken salads, mayonnaise, cucumbers, pickles, cabbage, tea, coffee, alcohol, pastry, too much sweets, and cheese if it disagrees.

Five to six light meals a day are preferable to three heavy meals.

The flow of gastric juices is constitutional, thus the regulation of digestion depends on the general vitality as well as on foods. The circulation must be forceful, the habit of deep breathing and of regular periods of complete rest of body and mind must be established.

Since one with chronic gastritis is liable to have many idiosyncrasies, he should not be urged to eat foods for which he has a dislike. The easily digested foods should be prepared in various ways and served in an appetizing, dainty manner.

There are four special phases of chronic gastritis: Mucous Gastritis, Hyperchlorhydria, Hypochlorhydria, and Achlorhydria.

In *Mucous Gastritis* there is a profuse secretion of mucus in the stomach. In this case it is always well to wash out the stomach before introducing food, as suggested above.

The same general diet suggested for acute gastritis should be followed.

The condition known as hyperchlor- **Hyperchlor-** hydria shows a liberal excess of hydro- **hydria** chloric acid. The condition is common, and is brought on by worry, nervous excitement, eating when overtired, irregularity of meals, imperfect mastication, and excessive use of alcohol.

The diet should be a mixed one, in about normal proportions. If anything, it should incline more to proteins than to starches.

The hydrochloric acid is necessary for the digestion of proteins and some physicians give a diet consisting almost entirely of proteins such as eggs, lean meat, etc., because hydrochloric acid reduces the protein to acid albumin, which is less irritating to the stomach than the free hydrochloric acid. However, the proteins are stimulating to the stomach and the protein proportion should not be carried to excess.

The best method is to follow a diet in which the foods have practically their normal balance—avoiding all irritating foods.

The juice of one-fourth of a lemon taken one-half hour before the meal will decrease the secretion of hydrochloric acid.

Limewater and milk may be used exclusively for two days; alkaline, effervescing mineral water may be used and then the diet should follow the general diet in chronic gastritis.

Hypochlorhydria is a diminution in the amount of hydrochloric acid. Since this acid is essential in gastric digestion of proteins, a decrease in its supply diminishes the power of the stomach to digest meat, eggs, etc. Physicians often administer hydrochloric acid about one hour after a meal. It should not immediately follow the meal consisting of part solid food, because it retards salivary digestion. Acid fruits, such as lemonade or egg lemonade, should be given half an hour after the meal instead of at the beginning.

Many advocate a diet omitting protein, but since protein foods stimulate the flow of gastric juices, they should *not* be omitted, but taken less freely. The meals should be at least six hours apart so as to allow time for digestion and to give the stomach rest.

Achlor-
hydria

When there is an entire absence of hydro-chloric acid, as in *achlorhydria*, the stomach, of course, cannot digest proteins and this digestion must be accomplished entirely by the trypsin of the pancreatic juice. The presence of liquefied protein, as beef juice in the stomach, however acts as a stimulus to the gastric juice and is an agency in again starting its flow.

The foods should be liquid, so as to pass through the stomach without irritating it. Clear milk must be excluded, because of the action of the rennin in coagulating the casein. This would irritate the stomach.

Pancreatinized milk (see page 99) may be used as an article of diet, also milk with limewater, junket, gelatin, cream, butter, bacon, olive oil, gruels, and any foods which will pass through the stomach without change and are digested by the pancreatic juice in the intestines.

Bran must be excluded from any cereals. Cereals or any carbohydrates cooked or masticated to a liquid state will pass through the stomach without difficulty and be digested and absorbed in the small intestine.

Dilatation results from continued over-eating (especially when the nerves are weak), or eating when overtired. The muscular walls become so weak that they fail to contract. Peristalsis is likewise weak, **Dilatation or Prolapsus of the Stomach** and the food, failing to digest promptly, ferments and forms gas. A dilated stomach is enlarged and its weight and weakness cause it to prolapse.

In the prolapsed condition the pyloric, or lower orifice of the stomach, is often nearly closed, partly by reason of its position and partly by the weakened folds of the stomach walls. Because of this obstruction to the free emptying of the contents into the duodenum, it is imperative that the food be of the simplest form, thoroughly masticated, and perhaps predigested and concentrated so as to be in as small an amount as possible. A chunk of food could not easily pass through the pylorus.

All liquid or semiliquid food should be subject to the chewing movements until it, also, is mixed with saliva. The stomach should not be overloaded with either food or water and for this reason six or more light meals a day, at regular intervals, is best.

A dilated stomach does not necessarily indicate that the digestive juices are not secreted in normal proportions, and easily digested proteins need not be avoided. It is desirable to furnish the proteins in concentrated form, as in meats, so as to get the most nutrition with the least bulk. They should be thoroughly masticated.

Milk may be used, with limewater, if sipped slowly and mixed with saliva.

Sugar should be used very sparingly, because it ferments readily and aggravates the distention. If it is evident that fermented products are in the stomach, it should be washed out with a stomach pump.

A tumor near the pylorus, or constriction of the pyloric orifice by prolapsus, will also cause dilatation of the stomach.

Beef juice, any of the better grades of meats, well masticated and containing no gristle, limewater and milk, soft-cooked eggs, and well-cooked cereals and vegetables should constitute the diet.

Avoid vegetables containing coarse fiber, fried foods, and freshly baked bread.

Liquid with the meal should be avoided, on account of the tendency to overload the stomach.

Cold water, taken a swallow at a time at intervals during the day, has a tonic effect on the relaxed muscles. It also incites the flow of gastric juice.

The best and quickest means of correcting a prolapsed and dilated stomach is by rest in bed for several weeks, with special exercises to raise the viscera and to strengthen all abdominal muscles, as well as the muscular coat of the stomach itself. The food must be given in small quantities every hour.

Ulcer of the Stomach   When this condition is severe, accompanied with severe pains and vomiting of blood, the nourishment is given through the rectum for from five to ten days. Then, for ten days, a milk diet with bouillon, barley water, a beaten egg, and once a day, after the third day, strained oatmeal gruel, is taken.

Limewater is added to the milk to avoid the formation of large curds and to neutralize the acids of the stomach. The patient is given half a cup of milk every hour for three days, from 7 A.M. to 9 P.M. From the third to the tenth day the quantity may be increased to one cupful, then to a cup and a half, and the periods between feedings lengthened to two hours. If the milk is thoroughly heated, but not boiled, before the limewater is added, it digests more readily.

After ten days, for the succeeding ten days the nourishment should be given every two hours and the diet varied by semiliquid foods, such as gruels, toast water, soft-boiled egg (once a day), beef juice, two softened crackers (once a day), gelatin, buttermilk, and strained soups. (See page 313, Semisolid Foods.)

After twenty days the patient, if all is well, may very gradually resume a normal diet, beginning with baked potatoes, softened toast, lamb chops, a small piece of steak or white meat of chicken. It is imperative that all food, liquid or solid, be thoroughly mixed with saliva and that solids be chewed to a pulp.

Liquids must not be swallowed either hot or cold, but about body temperature. Cold water may be taken into the mouth when more palatable than warm and held there until about body temperature before it is swallowed. All liquids should be sipped, not swallowed in gulps.

When the condition of ulcer has existed for some time complete rest in bed for from six to ten weeks is advisable. Either the diet suggested above or, if it is desired to gain in weight, a diet of milk, cream, and eggs may be followed. All solid food should be avoided.

[INTESTINAL DISORDERS

Most cases of intestinal difficulties may be traced to a clogged condition, either due to a weakness of the nerves and of the intestinal muscles, with resultant weak peristalsis, or to insufficient lubrication.

If the waste is not promptly moved through the intestines, irritation may result and the poisons from bacterial fermentation will be absorbed by the system.

Deranged digestion in the stomach also interferes with digestion in the intestines. Likewise delayed intestinal digestion affects digestion in the stomach.

Constipation   A large number of cases of constipation become chronic because of the failure to respond to Nature's call at a regular time each day. Many others are due to weakness of the muscular walls of the intestines or to the nerves controlling them. In this event the intestinal peristalsis is weak.

Constipation may be mechanical, due to obstruction of the intestine in some part of its course, *e. g.*, prolapsus, tumor, or a kink in the bowel itself.

Still another cause is a failure of the liver to discharge sufficient bile into the intestines to lubricate the feces.

Many chronic cases are due to the pill and drug habit. When one continues to take pills, the condition brings a result similar to the feeding of "predigested" food—if the work is done for the organs they become lazy and rely on artificial aid. *Every part of the body requires activity for strength.*

If the intestines are cramped by the clothing it may cause constipation by restraining their normal exercise during movements of the body in walking, etc. Exercises for the intestines should be taken morning and night.

Constipation may exist even when there apparently

is a daily movement of the bowels. Material may accumulate in the large intestine because only a part of the contents is discharged and may cause the unpleasant symptoms which accompany constipation.

It may arise from irregularity in meals, or from overeating, thus causing derangements of digestion from disturbance of the normal process.

Insufficient food may cause it, because the mass is not large enough to be acted on by the muscular movements of the intestines.

Too much strong tea, by its astringent action, lessens the secretions of mucus and causes the mass to become too dry.

Too little water may be taken and the food not sufficiently moistened; food may be concentrated and leave little residue.

Overeating, especially when the intestinal muscles are weak, furnishes a greater bulk than the intestines have the power to propel, hence a semi-paralysis and inactivity result.

Anxiety and grief or worry may inhibit the action of the nerves and thus cause a stagnation of movement on the part of the bowels.

The *cause* of the difficulty must be ascertained before relief can be gained.

The most natural relief for constipation, therefore, comes through exercise, particularly when directed to the muscles of the stomach and of the intestines and to the nerve centers controlling them.

The free use of water and such foods as figs and raisins, prunes, dates, grapes, apples, and rhubarb, which are laxative in effect, are helpful. These have best effect when eaten just before retiring or when the stomach is empty.

The use of vegetables which furnish a large bulk of fiber is often beneficial. Cabbage, celery, lettuce, spinach, mustard greens, oyster plant, and asparagus consist largely of residue. Onions are also laxative, especially when boiled. Tomatoes possess a special laxative effect for many individuals.

When derangements of digestion make raw fruits undesirable, they may be cooked and thus used for their laxative effect. They are not so laxative when cooked with much sugar, because much sugar may cause fermentation and gas. A little bicarbonate of soda added to acid fruits after cooking will correct the acidity and not so much sugar will be needed.

Two or three glasses of water should be taken on rising and before retiring. This cleanses the stomach as well as aids in relieving the dryness of the bowel contents.

Oatmeal, or any cereal containing the bran, is laxative. Such are bran or corn-meal bread, Boston brown bread made with molasses, and Graham bread.

Children should be trained to attend to Nature's call regularly *every* day. The best time is shortly after breakfast.

Enteritis   *Inflammation or Catarrh of the Intestines* is similar in its nature to Gastritis or Catarrh of the Stomach.

Acute Enteritis, or cholera morbus, is usually caused by a strong irritant—either by some food which disagrees, by unripe fruits, or by a mass of undigested food.

A fast of two or three days is the usual initial dietetic treatment.

A free drinking of water not only soothes the irritated intestines, but it cleanses the intestinal tract and assists in eliminating elements of fermentation; if these are not eliminated, they will be absorbed into the blood.

˝Absolute quiet in bed is necessary.

After the fast, a liquid and semiliquid diet is followed until inflammation is relieved and diarrhea and vomiting have ceased. Milk, strained gruels, broths, strained soups, buttermilk, eggs (soft cooked or raw), beef juice, barley water, custards, junket gelatins, soft puddings, etc., are most nourishing and cause little irritation. (See page 313, Semisolid Foods.)

Milk should be mixed with limewater to prevent the formation of large curds and should be sipped. Water should not be taken, as it tends to increase the diarrhea. Ice may be held in the mouth to relieve thirst.

All irritating foods, such as coarse vegetables, pickles, acid fruits and fruits with coarse seeds, candies, beer, wines, and salads must be omitted.

Chronic Enteritis has the same general cause as acute enteritis, though its onset is slow and it takes a correspondingly longer time to correct.

A milk diet for two or three weeks may be necessary to rest the bowels.

When food is taken, if undigested particles appear in the stool, it may be necessary to use predigested foods for a while.

If acute, dysentery demands complete rest in bed. The diet, in both acute and **Dysentery** chronic cases, must be confined to easily digested foods such as peptonized or pancreatinized milk (see pages 99 and 308), boiled milk, meat juice, and the white of egg, beaten and served with milk.

Blackberry brandy and tea made from wild cherry bark tend to check the inflammation.

During convalescence, care must be taken not to overfeed. Fruits and vegetables should be avoided. Begin a more liberal diet with an increased amount of beef juice, gradually adding tender beefsteak, roast beef, fish, white meat of chicken, eggs, custards, jelly, dry toast, blancmange, well-boiled rice, and other easily digested food. The beef and egg are particularly valuable, because of the anemia occasioned by the loss of blood.

DERANGEMENTS OF THE LIVER

The liver is not, in a strict sense, a digestive organ, but the digested food must pass through it and undergo certain chemical changes.

For a fuller understanding of the reasons for the following suggestions regarding diet in liver derangements, the chapter on the "Work of the Liver," pages 151–152 should be reread.

It will be recalled that the liver acts not only on the foods, but it also stands on guard to neutralize poisonous ferments, due to putrefactions absorbed from the intestines, and to render them harmless. To a limited extent it also oxidizes alcohol.

After the gorging of a heavy meal, the overloaded blood and liver express themselves in a sluggishness of the brain and one feels mentally as well as physically inert.

Since both carbohydrates and protein undergo chemical changes in the liver, it is evident that a diet consisting of an excess of either, must overwork the liver, not only through the nutritive food elements absorbed, but through the toxic substances which may be produced.

The regulation of diet, when the liver is in an abnormal condition, must be more in the *quantity* than in the *quality* of food.

The condition of the liver depends also on the activity of the intestines, since the poisonous products from imperfectly digested and fermenting food, not being eliminated, will be absorbed and carried to the liver. If the food remains in the intestines too long, it is attacked by the bacteria always present there, fermentation results and poisons are absorbed and carried to the liver, which usually can render them harmless to the system. If for any reason the liver is diseased, overloaded, or its action is sluggish, these toxins are absorbed in larger quantities than the liver is able to handle, hence they reënter the blood and poison the system.

The most important corrective agencies, when the liver is inactive, is a fast for a day or two, a free drinking of water, deep breathing, and exercise so directed as to bring a free supply of blood to this organ.

It is apparent that the blood must carry its full quota of oxygen to assist in eliminating both the nitrogenous waste and the poisons. It must also be remembered that the liver must oxidize the waste from its own tissues, as well as from other parts of the system.

This condition is due to the overproduction of bile which may be absorbed into **Biliousness** the blood to inactivity of the body and a resultant sluggish circulation of blood; to overwork of the liver due to overeating; and to insufficient breathing of pure air. It may also result from constipation and the resultant absorption of toxic matter, as previously described.

It may be occasioned also by obstruction of the opening of the bile duct into the intestines from an excess of mucus in the duodenum. In such cases exercises for the intestines are clearly indicated.

In the bending, twisting, and squirming movements which the infant in the cradle makes, the liver is regularly squeezed and relaxed. The same is true of the free movements of an active child at play. If during adult life these same free movements of bending and twisting the trunk were continued daily and correct habits of free breathing of pure air were established, there would be little call for "liver tonics."

The transformation of carbohydrates in the liver is an important part of its work and in case of inactive liver the sugars and starches should be limited in the diet. Protein stimulates the activity of the liver, yet it is a mistake to allow a diet too rich in protein. The best method is to cut down the quantity of food.

Two glasses of water an hour before breakfast, followed by brisk exercise for the vital organs and deep breathing, are the best remedies.

The daily action of the bowels is imperative.

In extreme cases a fast of two or three days, with a copious use of water, is recommended. Following this fast the diet should consist of easily digested foods, eliminating those containing starch and sugar in too great proportions, as bread, cereals, and potatoes. The amount should be as limited as is consistent with the actual necessity for rebuilding and for energy.

The taking of fats should be restricted in biliousness. The presence of fat in the duodenum stimulates the flow of pancreatic juice, which in turn stimulates the secretion of bile, thus overworking the liver.

Lemon stimulates the action of the gastric glands and thus tends to increase the liver activity.

It has been thought that eggs and milk cause sluggish liver action. There is no physiological reason for this if too much food is not eaten. The fact is often lost sight of that milk is a food as well as a beverage and that when milk constitutes an appreciable part of the diet other foods should be limited accordingly.

The DIET may be selected from the following:

Soups.—Light broths and vegetable soup with a little bread toasted in the oven.

Fish.—Raw oysters, fresh white fish.

Meats.—Mutton, lamb, chicken, or game.

Farinaceous.—Whole wheat or Graham bread and butter, toast buttered or dry, toasted crackers, cereals in small portions.

Vegetables.—Fresh vegetables, plain salads of watercress, lettuce, and celery, without oil or mayonnaise dressing. Lemon juice and salt may be used.

Desserts.—Gelatins, fruits, cornstarch, ice cream, junket, simple puddings,—all with *very little sugar.*

Liquids.—Hot water, lemonade, orangeade, toast water, buttermilk, loppered milk, and unfermented grape juice—not too sweet.

AVOID.—All rich, highly seasoned foods, candies, cheese, pies, pastry, pancakes, or any fried foods, salmon, herring, mackerel, bluefish, eels, dried fruits, nuts, and liquors of all kinds.

Gallstones occur most often in persons after middle life, especially in those of sedentary habits. **Gallstones**

A substance called cholesterin is normally present in solution in bile and in the tissues. When, through inactivity of the liver, or when because of sedentary habits the bile remains too long in the system, the cholesterin is precipitated, and, mixed with mucus, it forms gallstones.

A diet composed mostly of starch and fat favors their formation.

All dietetic measures should be combined with exercise to promote the flow of bile into the intestines.

Two glasses of hot water should be taken in the morning and before retiring. Several glasses of cold water should be drunk through the day.

Sweets and starches should be largely eliminated from the diet; sweet fruits and root vegetables must be avoided.

Fresh green vegetables and acid fruits may be taken. Potatoes contain calcium, but because they contain much more potassium, which lessens the liberation of calcium, they may also be used.

For foods rich in calcium which should be avoided see page 219.

Foods causing calcium oxalate deposits should be avoided as they may cause the formation of gallstones. For a list of these see p. 219.

Meat, if taken, must be lean and eaten only once a day. Beef and chicken are the preferable meats. Fresh fish may be used.

Alcohol must not be taken and coffee and tea must be limited in strength and quantity.

Active exercise must be practiced daily and full elimination secured from the bowels.

The person afflicted with gallstones must not sit too long or in a cramped position.

The presence of fat in the duodenum increases the flow of pancreatic juice which, in turn, stimulates the flow of bile, so olive oil is often recommended in case of gallstones. It is questionable whether it is of benefit, because, as stated, much fat upsets the liver.

Watch the water supply. Hard water which contains lime should be boiled to precipitate the calcium.

DERANGEMENTS OF THE KIDNEYS

The office of the kidneys is to eliminate from the system certain nitrogenous elements in solution; the work of the kidneys, in most conditions, is aided by copious drinking of water.

The influence exerted on the function of the excretory organs by the components of the food has not been given the attention it merits.

If the fluids are not taken in sufficient amount and much animal food is eaten, the urine becomes more concentrated and may irritate the kidneys or the bladder and give rise to calculi (kidney stones) or to the deposit of uric acid. Watery vegetables, juicy fruits, milk, water, and most beverages, by increasing the output of urine, lessen its acidity and density.

A diet limited to certain articles of food by the likes or dislikes of the individual, as the starches and sugars, too large consumption of acid fruits or too fatty foods may cause the appearance in the urine of abnormal amounts of various substances, as sugar, phosphates, calcium oxalate, or fatty acids.

Acid fruits in moderation aid digestion and favor suitable elimination, but when eaten to excess, as lemons, taken two or three or more a day by those striving to reduce flesh, the urine is increased in acidity, and irritation of the bladder may ensue.

Too great an amount of food tends to overwork the kidneys as well as the liver and various derangements result; these must be treated dietetically as well as by medicine.

In inflammation of the kidneys (nephritis), the secretion of urine is lessened or may cease.

Acute Nephritis The kidneys and digestive system must not be overworked and all food must be eliminated save milk until the kidney function is restored. It may be diluted with lime or Vichy, or skimmed milk or buttermilk may be used.

Water flushes the kidneys and if the urine increases in amount when water is given its use may be continued. When the amount of urine is diminished or the kidneys are not functioning at all, water, or any fluid or food that gives the kidneys work, must be given only on the advice of a physician, as serious harm may be done unless the inflamed kidneys are given as near perfect rest as possible. Sometimes even milk must be reduced to one pint a day.

In the event that the kidneys do not excrete, the pores of the skin must be kept freely open by sweat baths to assist in the elimination of urea.

Dr. Hall recommends a milk and cream diet of from three to seven pints a day, for a few days, according to the case—two parts of milk to one of cream. If the urine is scanty, he reduces it to one and one-half pints a day, taken in four or five installments. After the three to seven days of milk diet he gradually introduces starches and fats into the diet.

Bright's Disease This is an inflammatory condition of the kidneys in which albumin appears in the urine. It results from irritation and may be acute or chronic.

The appearance of albumin in the urine does not always indicate disease. It may be temporary, merely indicating that the diet, for the time being, is too heavy or contains an excess of protein, especially meat.

Several tests from one to two weeks apart are often necessary to determine whether the condition is merely temporary or is due to inefficient action of the kidneys.

When for any reason the kidneys have difficulty in eliminating the nitrogenous waste of the system, the dietitian must eliminate protein food as closely as may be consistent with the body necessities. Besides restricting the amount of nitrogenous foods, the kidneys must be assisted in eliminating the nitrogenous waste and the products of inflammation by a copious drinking of water, unless the kidneys are so inflamed that complete rest is indicated.

Hot water and hot drinks are best in the morning, such as toast water, barley water, cream of tartar, lemon and acid drinks. Unless a dropsical condition is present one may drink freely of cool water.

In acute cases the patient is put on a diet of from two to three pints of milk a day, given one-half pint every three or four hours, diluted with one-third as much hot water. Complete rest is imperative.

In chronic cases, exercise, judiciously directed to the extremities, particularly to the legs and the back, will do more than anything to aid the elimination of an excessive accumulation of fluid as in dropsy. This condition is usually accompanied by constipation and poor circulation, and exercises directed to the liver and bowels aid in carrying off the excess of fluid by way of the intestines; this will rest the kidneys. A cure requires patience and perseverance.

In chronic cases it is also well to follow a milk diet for a number of weeks. The quantity of milk for an exclusive milk diet must depend on the age and size of the patient as well as on his ability to exercise. If he is confined to his room, from ten to sixteen

18

glasses of milk a day are sufficient. If he is taking a great deal of exercise, he may take from eighteen to twenty glasses of milk a day. If he loses weight on the milk diet, bread and rice may be added, or potato soup, cereals, tapioca, and various gruels.

If the milk is not well borne, malted milk or pre-digested milk with butter and cream may be substituted. If the casein in the milk is not well digested, cheese must not be used. An egg once or twice a week and fruit and fresh vegetables may be given, but meat should be omitted.

A. F. Pattee gives the following diet in Bright's disease.

DIET

Soup.—Vegetable or fish soup, broths with rice or barley.

Fish.—Raw oysters or clams, fresh fish broiled or boiled.

Meats.—Eat sparingly, chicken, game, fat bacon, fat ham.

Farinaceous.—Stale bread, whole wheat bread, toast, milk toast, biscuits, macaroni, rice, cereals of all kinds.

Vegetables.—Onion, cauliflower, mashed potatoes, mush-rooms, lettuce, watercress, spinach, celery, cabbage.

Desserts.—Ripe raw fruits, stewed fruits, rice, tapioca, bread and milk puddings, junkets, cocoa.

Liquids.—Toast water, weak tea, pure water, peptonized milk, malted milk, fresh buttermilk, milk and hot water in equal parts, whey, unfermented grape juice.

AVOID.—Fried fish, corned beef, hashes, stews, pork, veal, heavy bread, batter cakes, lamb, mutton, beef, gravies, beans, peas, malt or spirituous liquors, tobacco, coffee, ice cream, cake, pastry.

This diet is tentative only and may be modified to suit the individual. If improvement is manifest after a month or two of the restricted diet, steak, roast beef, and eggs may be gradually added. If, when the urine is examined, the use of meat causes a return of albumin, it must be dropped.

In these cases, active outdoor exercise, full, deep breathing systematically practiced at intervals, a calm quiet attitude of mind and care not to overeat and to keep the bowels active will materially aid recovery.

Interference with the action of the kidneys is apt to result in a retention within the system of the elements which they, in normal condition, eliminate from the system—such as urea, uric acid, urates, sulphates, phosphates, etc. They are the result of the oxidation and the breaking down of the proteins of the body. If the kidneys do not eliminate these the result is a systemic poisoning, and the dietetic treatment must be such as will aid them to act freely.

Uremia or Uremic Poisoning

Fruits should be used freely. The citrus fruits (lemons, oranges, limes, etc.) are the best; they neutralize acids and promote the alkalinity of the blood.

When the system shows an excess of uric acid, the chances are that the individual has not been living on a diet containing too large a proportion of protein, but that he has been eating more than he requires of all kinds of foodstuffs. His system thus becomes weakened and he does not breathe deeply nor exercise sufficiently to oxidize and throw off the waste.

Meats, eggs, and legumes should be eliminated from the diet. A free drinking of water, milk with limewater, cereals, buttermilk, kumys, barley water, toast water, lemonade, orangeade, vegetables, and fruit should form the diet.

Exercise and free breathing of fresh air are imperative. All food should be thoroughly masticated.

Excess of Uric Acid When this condition appears it is due to too great an amount of animal or nitrogenous food. It causes dizziness, ringing in the ears, general nervousness, and insomnia.

Uric acid does not render the urine acid but when the acidity of the urine is increased, due to too much animal food, the tendency of the uric acid to form a crystalline deposit is increased. This deposit, as "gravel," may occasion attacks of renal colic or become the basis, when mixed with mucus, for kidney stones or stones in the bladder.

Headaches if due to uric acid will often cease when animal food is lessened.

Too much candy or sweet foods, or too much fat, eaten in connection with much protein, by deranging the liver function, change the character of the urine and favor the production of uric acid, causing such chronic ailments as bronchitis, asthma, severe nerve depression, gout, and neuralgia.

The natural relief is obtained by control of the diet, supplying less protein. One may either eliminate the proteins from the diet, or may cut down the entire quantity of food. Free elimination through a free action of the kidneys, the pores of the skin, and the lungs, is necessary.

Systematic exercise, deep breathing, copious drinking of water, and fresh air day and night, are the best aids. Exercise and deep breathing promote a free elimination of waste through the pores of the skin, and the free drinking of water creates a greater elimination through the kidneys, thus throwing off the excess of acid.

The skins of fruits contain various acids which favor the alkalinity of the blood. Therefore it is better, when there is an excess of uric acid, to eat unpeeled fruits. Apples, eaten raw and unpeeled, because of the acids, are of benefit. Citrus fruits, such as lemons, oranges, and grapefruit, are advised. Pears, and other sweet or bland fruits, because of the lack of acid, are less valuable.

Pea pods when young may be cooked with the peas. String beans, spinach, celery, and asparagus are of value.

All rich sauces and gravies must be avoided.

Osler remarks that "gout is evidence of an overfed, overworked, and consequently clogged machine."

Gout

It is usually the result of high living. It most often attacks people past middle age, who have indulged in large quantities of food, especially the nitrogenous foods which are not thoroughly oxidized due to sluggish circulation and shallow breathing. The process, imperfectly carried on, allows the accumulation of the waste material which cannot be excreted by the kidneys unless completely transformed by oxidation. These insoluble materials are deposited in the joints, act as irritants, and occasion the attacks of pain, swelling, and tenderness which usually mark the acute condition.

It is most common in those who habitually overeat, take little exercise, or who have frequently indulged in alcohol.

Sugar and fat in quantities are injurious as the oxidation of the protein is not carried on as completely when these are in excess. In fact, the entire system is more sluggish. Fat also interferes with gastric digestion as it passes through the stomach unchanged, and if the particles of food have a coat of the fat liquefied by the heat of the stomach, it is difficult for the gastric juice to exert its power.

The use of meat and sugars tends to make the urine acid and the use of vegetables favors its alkalinity, rendering it less acid. Therefore it becomes necessary to eliminate meat from the diet, to cut down the fats and carbohydrates, and to eat freely of fruits and vegetables.

Alcohol is absolutely prohibited.

In *acute cases* a diet of bread and milk, or toast and milk, with light vegetable broths, should be followed for from one to three days.

In *chronic cases* the diet may consist of the following:

Soups.—Vegetable broths.

Fish.—Fresh fish, shell fish, raw oysters.

Meats.—It is better to omit all meats. If meat is eaten at all, it should be confined to game, chicken, and fat bacon.

Farinaceous.—Cereals, crackers, dry toast, milk toast, macaroni, graham or whole wheat bread, rye bread, oatmeal, and any of the breakfast foods.

Vegetables.—Celery, lettuce, watercress, all greens, without vinegar, string beans, green peas, potatoes, carrots, and beets.

Fruits.—All fruits, stewed or fresh. Unpeeled apples are especially recommended. (Greens, without vinegar and unpeeled apples, increase the action of the kidneys.)

Desserts.—Plain puddings, junket, rice, stewed or fresh fruits.

Liquids.—Pure water, toast water, barley water, buttermilk, malted milk, milk.

Eat eggs sparingly, and in severe cases, not at all.

AVOID.—Alcohol, coffee, tobacco, dried fruits, nuts, cheese, candies, pastries, pies, spices, rich puddings, fried foods, vinegar, pickles, lemons, rhubarb, mushrooms, asparagus, sweet potatoes, tomatoes, gravies, patties, rich soups, lobster, salmon, crabs, mackerel, eel, veal, pork, goose, duck, turkey, salted, dried, potted, or preserved fish or meat (except bacon).

It is not sufficient to eliminate the foods to be avoided. To reduce the quantity of food is also necessary; yet this must be watched as the diet should not be so rigid as to cause a lowering of vitality. Eating between meals should not be allowed.

In an acute attack the diet should be confined to milk, vegetables, and fruits.

This is the result of a serious disturbance of nutrition. Since its presence is made **Diabetes** manifest by the appearance of sugar in the urine, it is considered among the derangements of the kidneys. However, one should not be apprehensive of diabetes if the urine test for a day shows sugar. This may be due to an excess of carbohydrates, particularly of sugar, in the diet a day or two previous and all trace of it may disappear in a day or two. If continued tests show an excess, nutritional disturbances are indicated. The treatment is almost entirely dietetic.

The most usual form of diabetes is *diabetes mellitus.* It is supposed to be due to a disturbance in the metabolism of sugar. It may be aided by defective pancreatic ferments, the lack throwing more work on the liver in the metabolism of sugar.

The difficulty which confronts the dietitian is to prescribe a diet restricting the carbohydrates which will keep up the body weight and not disturb the nutritive equilibrium. The patient has a craving for sugars and starches, but the system cannot make use of them, and the heat and energy must be supplied by fats.

The diet must consist largely of protein and fat. One danger lies in the tendency of acetic and other acids to accumulate in the blood, which affects the nervous system.

While, as a rule, the craving for certain foods is an indication that the system needs the elements contained in them, the desire of the diabetic patient for sugars and starches *must not* be indulged more than absolutely necessary, because of the inability of the system to utilize them.

There is often a distaste for fat, but its use is imperative when it is well borne, because the weight and general vitality must be maintained. If all carbohydrates are eliminated from the diet, the system will often suffer severely. Therefore the dietitian must determine the diet suited to the individual case, since complicated conditions may exist and the diet for one patient will work harm to another. The fleshy patient can stand a rigid diet, eliminating sugars and starches, much better than one who is thin and emaciated. A thin, weak patient often cannot endure too rigid a diet.

The following list of foods contain least carbohydrates: clear soup of meat without vegetables, all acid fruits, eggs, clams, and lobsters, fresh fish of all kinds, fresh meat of all kinds, and most smoked meat, olive oil, butter, peas, beans, all fresh vegetables (except carrots, parsnips, squash), onions, artichokes, cauliflower, cabbage, and asparagus.

Fats may be supplied in the yolks of eggs, cream, butter, cheese, bacon, and oily nuts, as butternuts, Brazil nuts, almonds, hazel nuts, walnuts, pecans; all should be well chewed.

In beginning a diet, the change must not be too sudden. Potatoes, when they agree, may be used in small quantities as a substitute for bread. At least a week's time should be allowed for the elimination of all sugar and starch. Begin by eliminating sugars and next bread, cereals, anything made with flour, and potatoes.

Sometimes it is necessary to begin with an all milk diet for a day or two.

Van Noorden gives the following diet, free from carbohydrates, which has been in general use in Europe and America.

Breakfast

Tea or coffee, 6 ounces.
Lean meat (beefsteak, mutton chop, or ham), 4 ounces.
Eggs, one or two.

Lunch

Cold roast beef, 6 ounces.
Celery, or cucumbers, or tomatoes with salad dressing.
Coffee, without milk or sugar, 2 ounces.

Dinner

Bouillon, 6 ounces.
Roast beef, 7½ ounces.
Green salad, 2 ounces.
Vinegar, 2½ drams.
Butter, 2½ drams.
Olive oil, 5 drams, or spinach with mayonnaise, large portion.

Supper, 9 P. M.

Two eggs, raw or cooked.

Van Noorden includes alcohol, in whisky, in his diet and most physicians follow the theory that alcohol aids in the digestion and absorption of fats; the need is recognized since fats must be supplied, yet the sweet wines and beers contain sugar while the sour wines contains acids, which may disturb digestion.

DERANGEMENTS OF LUNGS AND BRONCHI

Asthma   In this affection the free entrance of air into the lungs as well as its free exit is hampered by a condition of the bronchial muscles, the mucous membrane of the bronchi, and the muscles of the diaphragm. The muscles contract spasmodically without due or proper relaxation. This causes a congestion and swelling of the mucous membrane of the bronchi which still further hamper the ingress and egress of air.

Any digestive derangement which causes the formation of gas distends the stomach and intestines, interferes with the free action of the diaphragm, and prevents the free movement of the abdominal muscles.

The chemical action of the undigested and fermenting substances in the digestive tract irritates the nerves and may cause the spasm of the muscles. Digestive derangements will often cause the onset of an attack of asthma in those afflicted with this disorder.

The correction of the conditions in the stomach and intestinal tract will often ameliorate the attacks. Care must be taken not to overload the stomach and intestines, to eat easily digested foods which agree in the particular case. All food found to cause any digestive disturbance should be avoided.

Constipation must be remedied by gentle exercises and massage of the abdomen as free elimination removes material which might aid in inciting an attack.

Many asthmatics are comparatively comfortable during the day, the attacks coming on toward evening or during the night. In this case, the evening meal should be light and easily digested, the heavy meal being taken at noon.

Hot stuffy rooms increase the disorder and plenty of fresh air should be secured both by night and by day.

Many of these individuals make no exertion, fearing to bring on an attack.

Exercise, particularly of the lungs in breathing, should be gradual at first and be increased as improvement is shown. Exercises directed to expansion of the deeper cells of the lungs and to equalize the circulation throughout the entire system will call the excess of blood from the bronchial tubes and in many cases will cause the difficulty to disappear. A forceful, equalized circulation, with regulation of digestion, will do more for asthma than any known agency.

Derangements in digestion, common in this affection, are due to several conditions. **Tuberculosis**

The increased temperature is caused by the efforts of the system to counteract the poisons produced by the action of the bacillus. The increase in temperature in the stomach lessens the secretions and the peristaltic action, causing the food to ferment and to be vomited or to pass practically undigested into the intestine, thus throwing an excess of work on the intestinal secretions.

The bacilli-laden sputum, if swallowed, is apt to produce disorders of the stomach. This still further complicates the question of digestion.

Malnutrition, because of these derangements, increases the unfavorable outlook for the patient in this disease. Hence the diet, especially in chronic cases, is of great importance.

When means are ample, the question is much simplified, because by travel, change of scene, and pleasant surroundings the appetite is stimulated and greater variety in the diet can be gained. For those in moderate circumstances, save when free sanatoriums exist for the care of the tuberculous, it is most difficult to keep the diet from becoming monotonous and wearisome.

The appetite, especially in young people, is apt to be capricious, and it is important that the food be served daintily to tempt the patient to eat.

Growing children crave sweets and as these furnish energy they may be allowed to tuberculous children, in moderation, if they seem to be well assimilated. Any interference with digestion, however, must be guarded against.

It is better to give food in smaller quantities and oftener in order to guard against disturbed digestion from overloading the stomach. For this reason also it is better to give the heartiest food during the forenoon when the temperature is lowest.

Milk, butter, cream, olive oil, bacon, and cod-liver oil furnish the fat needed by the system in the most easily digested form and should be taken freely, if there is no irritation in the stomach which will prevent their assimilation. Variation in their use will often secure greater tolerance.

In chronic cases in which there is little or no fever, the fats are generally well assimilated and are beneficial.

The disease causes great wasting, and fats are especially important in counteracting this tendency. They may be given in alternation or be omitted from the diet for a day or two to avoid turning the patient against them.

If diarrhea exists fats must be given guardedly and if fats produce diarrhea they must be lessened or omitted until the diarrhea is controlled.

If one gains in flesh the chances are very strong that the case has been wrongly diagnosed, or that the disease, if present, is being overcome.

Milk, when it agrees, should form a large part of the diet. A glass may be taken with meals and two glasses between meals. The milk should be sipped slowly; lime water or carbonated water may be added to aid milk digestion.

Buttermilk, made by means of buttermilk tablets, from milk from which the cream has not been removed, or buttermilk mixed with one-fourth cream, kumys, or cream and water, if relished, may take the place of milk.

Eggs are also important aids in the diet, especially the yolk, because of the fat and iron it contains. If they disagree they may be taken with a few drops of lemon juice, orange juice, or grape juice, as these partially digest the egg.

The beaten and strained whites are very easily digested, and in that form may be taken in quantity of from six to twelve a day.

Tender, juicy meats, especially beef and mutton, may be taken, also meat juices and beef soups.

Highly seasoned foods should be avoided.

Fresh fish, clams, and oysters are permissible. Cereals, especially the coarse ones, that stimulate the bowel movements, if constipation exists, are valuable; oatmeal, rice, and corn-meal mush are especially good; also Graham or bran bread, and zwieback made with bran. If there is diarrhea bran should not be used.

Easily digested vegetables are of value, especially if cooked in little water so that most of the salts and other nutrients, which are so frequently boiled out of the vegetable, are retained. Baked apples or raw fruits, especially oranges, may be taken the first thing in the morning, or used as a dessert. Grapes, peaches, and other fruits in season may be taken in moderation.

Tea and coffee are best omitted.

The following constitutes a typical menu in ordinary cases. It must be varied to suit the individual case.

Breakfast:	Fruit, cereal, two eggs (poached or boiled) with or without a few slices of bacon; two slices of toast or bread, one-half ounce of butter, and a glass of milk.
10 a. m.:	Two or three eggs beaten in a glass of milk.
Luncheon:	Fish, chop, or steak, or some tender meat, one-half ounce of butter, one or two slices of bread, baked potato, or a dish of rice or hominy, green vegetables, or a salad of lettuce or tomato with olive oil, a dessert of custard or junket or some other nutritious dish, and a glass of milk.
3 p. m.:	Milk and eggs, meat broth and egg, milk and egg custard, or Graham crackers and milk.
Dinner:	Soup if desired, a glass of milk, a liberal helping of some special meat, roast beef, lamb, or mutton, chicken or turkey, potatoes, or a farinaceous vegetable, and a green vegetable, dessert, and a small piece of cheese.

This menu approximates the number of calories desirable in cases of tuberculosis that have not advanced to a stage in which complete rest is necessary. In that case a liquid or semiliquid diet is given.

When it is necessary that the diet be less expensive, beans, lentils, and eggs may take the place of meat at some meals, and oleomargarine may be substituted for butter. Milk and eggs, however, in the quantity advised, should be taken if possible.

If signs of overfeeding appear, due to the lessened activity of the digestive organs, shown by biliousness, coated tongue, etc., the food may be lessened in quantity until the condition is corrected.

If the tongue becomes coated the mouth should receive the care directed on page 95.

In all cases of weak lungs and chronic lung trouble, the diet should consist of easily digested foods. Those that cause flatulence should be avoided, as the distended stomach presses on the diaphragm and interferes with proper breathing and with the heart action.

DERANGEMENTS OF THE NERVES

No disturbance in any part of the body requires less medicine than a disturbance in the nerves. The correction must come through general hygienic treatment and directing the mind to optimistic thoughts.

Regular exercise, alternated with regular rest periods, the formation of the habit of complete nerve relaxation, the general regulation of an easily digested, nutritious diet, with deep breathing exercises, are the best remedies. The patient should be out of doors as much as possible and, unless too weak, should be employed at light work for mental diversion.

In cases of Neurasthenia, or "tired nerves," all vital organs are more or less affected, because the nerves do not properly **Neurasthenia** direct digestion, absorption, assimilation, or elimination.

The excessive use of stimulants, tea, coffee, or

alcohol, is often an exciting cause, because of over-stimulation of an already exhausted nervous system.

Complete rest of body and mind must be secured.

The diet should be light and of easily digested foods, but must be nutritious and taken regularly and systematically. Each case needs individual treatment, and the diet must be that most easily assimilated by the individual.

A free, correct breathing of fresh air, day and night, is imperative.

It is important also to thoroughly masticate all food and drink freely of water.

A change of thought, induced by a change of scene or companions, is helpful.

One of the most essential treatments of neurasthenia is to surround the patient with love and tenderness, but the patient should be led to avoid self-pity. This sets up a disagreeable trend of thought which relaxes nerve and vital forces and disturbs nutrition. Sympathy, good cheer, and an attitude of courageous optimism are the best nerve tonics.

Due to the weakened condition of the nerves, troubles which at other times seem trifles are as mountains and very real. Patience and intelligent sympathy, not apparent pity, are the best of medicines.

The tone of the nervous system is quickly altered by the state of mind of the individual. The reaction is a double one, constituting a "vicious circle." The nerves, disordered from worry, excessive fatigue, or other drains on the vitality, as a persistent pessimistic outlook on life, do not stimulate the natural digestive processes. The faulty digestion may fail to prepare a sufficient amount of food for use by the system. The nerves are thus underfed, which still further increases their inability to send motor and secretory impulses to the digestive and eliminative organs. Emaciation, general debility, and anemia may result.

Hence the importance, in the relief of any nervous condition, to see first that the attitude of mind be calm and quiet with the substitution of thoughts of hope and cheer for those of gloom and depression. The afflicted one must make a brave struggle because the tired body affects his thoughts as well as his thoughts his body.

There is no one food or set of foods which directly affect any nervous trouble unless this trouble be localized by disturbance in some particular organ. Then the effort must be to correct the difficulty in that organ.

Rest is imperative.

If thin, a fat-building diet should be followed to store energy-building reserve in the nerve centers.

In many cases of nerve debility the nerves seem to be stronger in the latter part of the day. When this is the case the hearty meal should be eaten at this time.

The condition of the blood is affected by the lack of its necessary ingredients, which **Neuralgia** may occur through faulty digestion as well as through improper diet. The resultant anemia of the nerves may produce neuralgic pains in any one or several of the tissues and organs, as the stomach, the intestines, the muscles, or the liver, etc. Neuralgia of the liver is sometimes mistaken for gallstone colic.

When underlying conditions of disease have been excluded by means of careful tests of the urine and blood, the diet becomes of importance and may result in the disappearance of the pain.

These pains occur chiefly in those who take little exercise and use improper food, which does not give the correct proportion of the needed elements to the system.

Exercise, as the body is usually weak, should be begun moderately but as soon as possible be made brisk and active to stimulate the vital organs to a more perfect performance of their function.

Plenty of oxygen must be secured by day and night and thorough elimination be maintained.

The diet must be nutritious and richer than is ordinarily taken. Milk, butter, cream, bacon, olive oil, and all fatty food should be freely used if assimilated. Beefsteak, roast beef, fresh vegetables, and eggs are valuable. Cocoa or chocolate, a glass of milk with a beaten egg, or a cup of broth into which an egg has been beaten may be regularly taken between meals.

If the digestion is feeble, light foods should first be taken and increased as the system becomes able to assimilate more hearty food.

Coffee, tea, highly spiced foods, alcohol, fried food, rich pastry, and much candy or sweet stuffs should be avoided.

Pain referred to the liver, if not caused by gallstones, usually indicates overwork of that organ, and fats, sweets, and starches should be avoided to give the liver rest.

Pain referred to the stomach is often caused by tobacco smoking or improper food, as too much candy or preserves, or too strong tea or coffee. Attention to the diet will usually relieve this variety of pain. If the pain comes on when the stomach is empty, due to a disorder of the nerves, the food should be lessened in quantity, be light, easily digested, and taken at shorter intervals.

Many conditions of the system due to dietetic errors which result in impoverished blood are accompanied by pains in the stomach. These are often neuralgic.

Poor assimilation of foods or indigestion produces pain because the tone of the nervous system is affected from the poor blood.

Neuralgia of the stomach often occurs in anemic conditions associated with constipation. In these cases a good, nutritious, but easily digested diet and better elimination will often cure, but as the changes in the blood and nerves are slow, one must be patient and persistent.

There is no better nerve tonic than pure air, exercise, cheerful thoughts, and rest.

Sweets, fried food, rich sauces, pastry, and highly seasoned food should be avoided.

When neuralgia of the stomach, due to an underlying condition such as rheumatism, gout, or diabetes occurs, the diet appropriate to the condition will often affect the cure of the neuralgia.

Chorea

The diet is of the greatest importance in this difficulty, as it is usually accompanied by anemia. Rest and a very nourishing and easily digested diet are essential. Sometimes a complete rest in bed and a milk diet, or a diet composed largely of milk, is the best means of treatment.

If possible the patient should be isolated and in the care of a trained nurse who is naturally cheerful and bright.

Children are especially liable to this malady. They are usually anemic and care should be exercised that they be not overworked in school and that they retire early and get from ten to twelve hours' sleep.

Their eyes must be kept from strain and the nervous system not allowed to become tense from too much excitement, as teasing by playmates or the family, etc.

They should be given the diet for Anemia on page 249.

DIET IN SKIN DISEASES

An improper diet or a lowered nerve tone are often shown by the condition of the skin.

When the waste of the system is not being properly eliminated through the other excretory organs the skin is required to throw off more than its normal amount.

The muddy complexion in biliousness or the congestion of the facial capillaries in the alcoholic are familiar examples.

Overeating, especially of food too rich or too concentrated, causes fermentation from non-digestion, or imperfect oxidation, due to too large an amount of nutriment for the amount of oxygen furnished to the tissues.

An inactive skin results in an accumulation of fat in the sebaceous glands with clogging of the ducts; germ infection in these clogged glands often results in pimples and boils. An excess of acid in the secretion of the sweat glands irritates the skin and causes eruptions.[1]

Chronic skin troubles are always increased and

[1] For treatment of pimples, see *Let's Be Healthy*, by Susanna Cocroft.

made more troublesome when there are errors in the diet, and they are often benefited and in some cases cured when the dietetic errors are corrected.

Skin troubles often occur when for any reason the nervous system is run down, because the weakened nerves cause the tissues or organs they supply to become inactive. The skin thus becomes affected with the rest of the body and derangements of its function appear. Increasing nerve tone will result in a disappearance of the skin disorders. This takes time.

All rich food and highly seasoned preparations, veal, pork, tea, coffee, pastry, too much sweets and fats, and any fruits and vegetables that cause flatulence should be avoided.

A diet of fruit, water, and Graham bread for three or four days, every week or two, daily exercise and deep breathing of pure air will usually clear the skin.

The skin of the face is materially cleared by the use of facial exercises which promote its activity and the elimination of waste. Exercises for increasing the tone of the skin and the muscles are as essential for the face as for the body.

In all skin troubles alcohol must be prohibited.

This is characterized by distressing itch- **Urticaria**
ing and may be caused by any article of **(Hives)**
food which disagrees. A more or less
irritant food or one difficult of digestion, such as strawberries, shellfish, pork, cheese, and sausage, are the foods which most usually produce it, if taken into an inactive stomach. When the intestines are in a sluggish condition the stomach does not act well, and

any food which does not digest promptly is liable to excite an attack.

It is remedied, by eating very lightly, by fasting for a day or two, by drinking *much* water, exercising, breathing deeply, and securing activity of the bowels. Care must be taken to avoid foods known to disagree.

Eczema The cause of this disorder is often difficult to ascertain, but it is aggravated or relapses occur when too much or too rich food is eaten. The skin is not able to dispose of all the material sent to it.

It often occurs in those who are excessive eaters of meat.

The diet may have to be confined to fruit, bread and milk, or crackers and milk for a few weeks.

Meat, if allowed, should be taken sparingly and not oftener than once a day—better only every other day. Beef and chicken are the preferable meats. If no improvement occurs, or if it be slight, meat should be omitted altogether. Eggs may be substituted for meat. A little fresh fruit, if thoroughly ripe, may be taken, but all made desserts must be avoided and very little sweets used. Cracked wheat, or other wheat cereal, with a little cream, may be eaten.

Oatmeal may provoke an attack because of the amount of fat in it. Foods may cause an attack in one case that have no detrimental action in another.

Skin eruptions, eczema-like, often occur if for any reason the diet has been too limited, as in the semi-starvation seen in poor children. In these cases a more nutritious diet will often cure.

Bananas, apples, cabbage, or fried foods, often cause a temporary attack or aggravate an existing condition.

The food must be thoroughly masticated, must be

taken at regular times, and not in excess. As this condition sometimes accompanies other diseases, any underlying condition must be sought, but all diet should be as simple as the needs of the system will bear. The foods which are found to increase the irritation of the skin are the ones to be avoided in each case.

The all-prevalent American habit of eating fried food often produces an intense itching of the skin in various parts of the **Pruritus (Itching)** body. It occurs often in those who eat food highly seasoned with pepper or other condiments. The articles of food causing the overstimulation must be avoided, and all fried food, pastries, or food containing much fat, must be greatly lessened or omitted altogether.

Itching is sometimes caused during the change of seasons due to the effect of the changing temperature on the nerves of the skin. To rub the skin with oil for two or three days to soften the dead cells and to aid their removal from the surface will secure a better circulation in the skin and help to eliminate the cause of the itching. A free drinking of water, fresh air, and exercise will help the condition.

The rapidly changing system of the growing boy and girl is especially liable to **Acne** disorders, due to improper eating, irregular habits, worry, lack of rest, or improper food. Eruptions, especially on the face, appear as a result. The sebaceous glands are especially active, and any alteration in the structure of the blood, due to deranged digestive processes and defective elimination by the skin, causes too great an amount of deposit in the fat glands. Their contents become hardened and infected by germs, with consequent irritation and reddening, and the condition known as acne is the result.

Once well established it is difficult to cure, but it often rapidly improves under a simple diet, rested nerves, cheerful, kind thoughts, and better digestion and elimination.

The food should be thoroughly masticated. Young people are prone to eat too hastily, and thus not thoroughly mix the food with saliva. If careful attention is paid to mastication of the food, water at meals is an aid to digestion. Water should be taken freely between meals, on rising and before retiring, for its diuretic and laxative effect.

All candy, and sweets, hot breads, corn bread, pastry, soups with much fat, rich hashes and sauces, fried food, pork, and veal should be eliminated from the diet.

A badly blotched face is an embarrassment, and no restriction in the diet should be deemed a hardship as a means to an improved digestion, increased mental vigor, and improved health.

A pimple on the face should be treated as antiseptically as a boil. The pus from a pimple which has "come to a head" should not be allowed to infect the surrounding skin. Infection may take place from towels or wash cloths used by one afflicted with acne. Care should be exercised to sterilize the surrounding skin by peroxide of hydrogen or alcohol before a pimple is opened and its contents should be taken up with absorbent cotton. A pimple should never be severely squeezed as the skin will be irritated and other pimples may result.

Often the infection from one pimple is spread by the

hands or by the wash cloth. Care should be taken to avoid this.

Exercise directed to the facial muscles and to the liver and digestive organs, deep breathing, plenty of oxygen by night and day, wholesome thoughts, plenty of sleep, and simple food, will eliminate or improve most skin difficulties. Care should be taken, by frequent bathing and friction baths, to aid the eliminative work of the skin.

Since the medical profession is unable to determine just what rheumatism is, it is **Rheumatism** difficult to prescribe a diet. The theory so long believed that it is caused by an excess of uric acid in the system is no longer held by most of the advanced physicians. Uric acid, however, sometimes accompanies the disease.

Some authorities hold that it is a nerve difficulty; others that it is caused by an excess of lactic acid; others hold that it is caused by infection from the tonsils and the gums.

Assuming that it is due to the failure of the system to promptly eliminate its waste, whether this failure to eliminate be through a weakened condition of the nerves, and the consequent failure to properly direct the body activities, the correction of the difficulty must lie in building up the general vitality and in aiding the system in its elimination.

Hot sweat baths, a free use of water, and a free use of fruits and fruit juices, particularly the citrus fruits, such as lemons, oranges, limes, etc., are desirable in moderation, because they increase the alkalinity of the blood, and because of their diuretic effect. Lemonade, orangeade, and all fresh fruits and vegetables are diuretic.

The diet should be cut down in quantity. If an excess of uric acid exists, meat may be eliminated and the suggestions given in the diet for Gout may be followed.

The food must be plain and well cooked, not highly seasoned, and the amount must be confined to the needs of the system as shown by the general condition.

Regular exercise, until the body is thoroughly heated, deep breathing of pure air day and night, and a copious drinking of water are necessary.

Leanness No definite diet can be given here for flesh building, because a lack of sufficient fat to round out the figure is due to faulty digestion or assimilation.

It may be that the strength of the muscles and nerves of the stomach, liver, and intestines should be built up by exercises and deep breathing, and it may be that the habit of nerve relaxation must be established. When the nerves are tense much nourishment is consumed in nervous energy and the nerves to the digestive organs and muscles being disordered, they interfere with digestion and assimilation.

It is apparent that the cause of the lack of flesh must first be corrected. Merely to give a fat-building diet may overload deranged digestive organs with sugars, starches, and fats, further weakening them.

Often leanness is due to inability to digest the starches or sugars, and when this is the case the condition must be remedied by strengthening the digestive organs through exercises for the muscles of the stomach and intestines, exercises to create a free activity of the liver and to strengthen the nerves controlling digestion. Deep breathing habits to insure sufficient oxygen to put the waste in condition for elimination are necessary. Most often sufficient food is eaten, but due to nerve tension or to sluggish circulation, particularly through the vital organs, it is not assimilated.

Usually, however, bodily flesh may be increased by increasing the liquids and the carbohydrate consumption and also the fat if these are assimilated.

If habits of life, overwork, improper food, unhealthy thoughts, nerve exhaustion, excessive nerve tension, or disease are responsible, they must first be corrected. Often the nerve tension must be relaxed by change of habit of both body and mind before the flesh will accumulate.

There must be no mental strain, and plenty of sleep must be secured.

If they can be assimilated, the diet should contain soups, butter, milk, cream, cocoa, chocolate, well-cooked cereals, as oatmeal, bread, tapioca, or rice puddings with cream and sugar, bread, potatoes, leguminous foods, as peas and beans, cake, honey, especially sweet fruits, carrots, parsnips, and other vegetables; meat not oftener than once a day.

Vinegar and too much spice, pastry, coffee, and tea should be avoided.

The free drinking of liquid is most important.

Obesity is caused by a disturbed balance of nutrition occasioned, often, by more food **_Obesity** being taken than the body requires. The resultant fat is deposited in and among the tissues.

It is most often seen in those in middle life of sedentary habit who continue to eat as heartily as ever without using a little thought to determine the actual body needs for food.

An excess of fat is often seen in light eaters, however. This is usually due to a weakness of nerve tissue, which does not direct the regular activities of the body—digestion assimilation, elimination, etc.—with sufficient force to burn up the normal amount of fat in automatic activities.

In all cases breathing is usually faulty, oxidation is incomplete, and little exercise for the vital organs is taken. Anemia may exist in such individuals.

The body fat is formed from various elements in foods, and a food which may cause obesity in one individual may not produce it in another. Fat meats, alcoholic drinks, or the excessive use of starches and sugars may cause it. The food at fault in each case must be determined and largely reduced or eliminated from the diet.

Many obesity cures are in existence, and have had considerable vogue from time to time. Anti-fat remedies are dangerous, as they lower the vitality of the system and render it liable to be attacked by disease. All such remedies act by decreasing the appetite and causing impairment of the digestion.

The rational method is to limit both the amount of food and the liquid to be taken, to increase oxidation by deep breathing and exercise. By restricting the carbohydrates and fats consumed the body calls on that stored in the tissues. In obesity, unless there is an underlying condition of disease, the amount of water should be limited while reducing and none should be drunk with the meals. Soup, milk, and all juicy fruits and all foods made from cereals should be taken sparingly; sugar must usually be forbidden and fat in the food limited to a little butter. One need not starve under this treatment for the diet may be varied enough to prevent monotony even though restricted.

Fresh green vegetables, fruit, and lean meat should form the main ingredients of the diet, but if gastric disturbances arise the diet must be varied to correct them. Meat should be eaten but once a day.

Extremes in diet should be strictly avoided; a sudden restriction of diet produces changes in the blood which may do harm. For this reason the amount of food taken should be gradually but steadily reduced and one article after another eliminated until the system becomes accustomed to the reduction.

Thorough elimination must be secured through exercise and deep breathing.

All alcoholic liquors must be omitted.

All diets for obesity must be prescribed for the individual condition. A diet suited to one person may be entirely unsuited to another. For this reason, and because of the danger of one following a diet which may be unsuited to the condition, diets for obesity are not given here.

Exercise and deep breathing must constitute an appreciable part of reduction methods to cause a combustion of the fat liberated. These are the natural, scientific means of reduction.

If one reduces by diet alone the excess of fat may not come from the part desired. One is likely to show the results first in the face and neck. One should exercise the parts desired to be reduced so as to oxidize the fat stored about these particular tissues.

A large number of the obese are afflicted with rheumatism, sluggish livers, sluggish action of the intestines, and weak nerves, and the diet must be governed accordingly.

The regulation of food for reduction of flesh must also be governed by age, sex, by the manner of breathing, and by the amount of daily exercise. The food must be regulated in accordance with the quantity of carbohydrates and fats daily consumed in heat and energy.

A rational study of the needs of the system and a persistent following of the indicated regimen will result in a steady reduction, renewed vitality, and a sense of "being fit." The better elimination secured by exercise and increased oxygen will aid the muscles to release the fat which may have caused them to become flabby.

Reduction must not be accomplished too suddenly, but it can be gained by a little self-denial and determination.

One who carries too much fat is much more liable to gout, rheumatism, apoplexy, high blood pressure, asthma, and bronchial affections.

Feeding the Convalescent When an individual is recovering from an illness the appetite often becomes excessively active, and his demands for food, if yielded to by the family or attendant, may produce digestive derangements from which recovery is slow.

On the other hand, too much food is often urged on the convalescent from a mistaken idea that large quantities of food are necessary in order to rebuild the enfeebled system.

Care must be taken not to return too rapidly to a solid diet when a liquid diet has been followed for some time. The digestive system shares in the general weakness and must not be overloaded.

The more easily digested foods, as ice cream, milk, tapioca, crackers and cream or cream toast, cream soups and meat broths thickened with bread crumbs rolled from toasted bread, custards, stewed fruits, corn meal, mush, in some conditions, cornstarch blanc-mange, boiled rice, and poached eggs may be given.

Later, when meat is added to the diet it should be scraped or finely minced so as to give the stomach as little work as possible until it regains its tone.

Potatoes, if allowed, should be baked or mashed.

Sweetbreads in cream, sponge cake or lady fingers with light cream may also be allowed.

At least a week should be taken in returning to a solid diet and the orders of the physician must be strictly followed. Pickles, nuts, or solid meats should not be allowed. They will often occasion a return of fever and possibly a relapse.

After typhoid fever or other lingering illness, the appetite is usually much increased, but great care must be exercised not to allow solid food before the condition of the stomach and intestines shows that danger is past. It is usual not to allow solid food in typhoid fever for two weeks after the fever has disappeared.

It is possible to make great variety in the diet even if it be light and easily digested and common sense must govern in the kind as well as the quantity of food allowed the convalescent.

Scraped beef or scraped chicken may be seasoned, lightly pan broiled, and made into a sandwich. The first solid meat may be creamed sweetbread, a bit of broiled tenderloin steak, or breast of chicken.

It is better to give small amounts both because of

the lessened work of digestion and because large amounts of food often destroy rather than aid the appetite.

If the appetite is capricious, or lacking, it needs to be stimulated by food appetizingly prepared and daintily served. A sloppy tray with half-cold tea or coffee will often cause complete loss of appetite.

The face and hands of an invalid should always be bathed before a meal; the fresh feeling induced is often an aid to the appetite. The mouth should be carefully cleansed after eating in order that no fermenting food particles may be carried into the stomach to cause disturbance there. Swabbing the mouth with cotton dipped in an alkaline wash or rinsing the mouth with listerine and water or peroxide of hydrogen and water will add greatly to the comfort of the sick, especially when the tongue is coated and the mouth bitter.

Great care should be taken not to allow bread crumbs to fall into or under the bedclothes, as a small bread crumb is often a source of great discomfort. The skin is especially sensitive and a small bread crumb may so disturb the mind as to cause a patient, otherwise doing well, to become restless and disturbed.

The invalid frequently forgets to ask for water and the attendant should see that a sufficient amount of water is taken. A glass of water should be placed where it is within easy reach and it should not be allowed to become warm. Cool water is one of the prime requisites in the invalid's dietary.

CHAPTER XI

THE purpose is not to give such recipes as are found in ordinary cookbooks, but simply to suggest foods useful for invalids, for semi-invalids, or for chronic, abnormal conditions of digestive organs.

Water. Pure and carbonated; mineral waters containing iron, sulphur, lithium, etc.

Hot drinks should be served at a temperature of from 122 to 140 degrees F. When water is used as a hot drink it should be freshly drawn, brought to a boil, and used at once. This sterilizes and develops a better flavor.

Cold water should be thoroughly cooled, but not iced, unless ice water is sipped very slowly and held in the mouth until the chill is off. Water is best cooled by placing the receptacle on ice rather than by putting ice in the water.

Fruit Juices. Under fruit juices are: grape juice, apple juice, currant juice, pineapple juice, orangeade, and lemonade.

They are especially grateful to fever patients and are often used to stimulate the appetite. They are particularly valuable for the acids which they contain, which aid the action of the kidneys and the peristaltic action of the digestive tract; they also increase the alkalinity of the blood.

Apples contain malic acid, lemons citric acid, and grapes tartaric acid. The ferment in the ripe pineapple juice aids in the digestion of proteins.[o]

Lemonade. Wash and wipe a lemon. Cut a slice from the middle into two pieces to be used in the garnish before serving; then squeeze the juice of the rest of the lemon into a bowl, keeping back the seeds. Add sugar and boiling water; cover and put on ice to cool; strain and pour into a glass.

Fruit Lemonade. To change and vary the flavor, fresh fruit of all kinds may be added to strong lemonade, using boiling water as directed above.

Egg Lemonade. Beat an egg thoroughly, add 2 tablespoonfuls of sugar, 2 tablespoonfuls of lemon juice, and gradually pour in one cup of cold water. Stir until smooth and well mixed. Serve thoroughly cold. This drink is very easily digested, the lemon having partly digested the egg; 2 tablespoonfuls of sherry or port may be added.

Bran Lemonade. Mix one-quarter cup of wheat bran with 2 cups of cold water. Allow this to stand overnight and in the morning add the juice of a lemon.

Pineapple Lemonade. Mix one-half cup of grated pineapple with the juice of 1 lemon and 2 tablespoonfuls of sugar; add one-half cup of boiling water, put on ice until cool, then add 1 cup of ice-cold water. Strain and serve.

Grape Lemonade. To 1 cup of lemonade, made as directed above, rather sweet, add one-half cup of grape juice.

Effervescing Lemonade. To the juice of 1 large lemon add a lump or two of sugar which has been rubbed on the rind. Pour on it half a pint of cold or ice water. Add half a teaspoonful of bicarbonate of soda after it has been placed in the tumbler.

Orangeade. One orange, 1 teaspoonful of sugar, three-quarters of a coffee cup of water. Wash and wipe the orange. Squeeze the juice into the sugar. Add the cold water which has previously been boiled. Strain.

Apple Water. Slice 1 pound of apples, put in a jar with one.

---

[1] Many of the recipes given for fruit beverages are adapted from *Practical Dietetics* by Alida Frances Pattee, Publisher, Mt. Vernon, N. Y.

fourth of a pound of brown sugar. Pour over apples and sugar 1 gallon of boiling water. When cool put the apples through a colander. Bottle but do not cork. Keep in a cool place. May be poured over toasted bread.

Mixed Fruit Drink. Mix one-quarter cup of grated pineapple, the juice of half a lemon, the juice of half an orange, 1 cup of boiling water, and sugar to taste. Put on the ice until cool. Strain and add more cold water and sugar according to taste.

Pineapple Juice. Pour one-half cup of pineapple juice over crushed ice and serve in a dainty glass. This is especially helpful in cases of weak digestion and in some throat troubles—as stated above, the pineapple aids protein digestion.

Lemon Whey. Heat 1 cup of milk in a small saucepan, over hot water, or in a double boiler. Add 2 tablespoonfuls of lemon juice; cook without stirring until the whey separates. Strain through cheesecloth and add two teaspoonfuls of sugar. Serve hot or cold. Garnish with small pieces of lemon.

Wine Whey may be made in the same way, using one-quarter cup of sherry wine to 1 cup of hot milk.

Grape Juice, Apple Juice, and Currant Juice are tonics and make a dainty variety for the sick room. They should be used according to their strength, usually about one-third juice to two-thirds water. They should be kept cold and tightly corked until ready to serve.

Grape Lithia. Add 4 ounces of Lithia-water to 1 ounce of grape juice and 2 teaspoonfuls of sugar.

Grape Nectar. Boil together 1 pound of sugar and one-half pint of water until it begins to thread. Remove from the fire and when cool add the juice of 6 lemons and 1 quart of grape juice. Let stand overnight. Serve with ice water, Apollinaris, or plain soda water.

Tea Punch. Pour boiling lemonade, sweetened to taste, over tea leaves. Allow the liquid to stand until cool. Then strain and serve with shaved ice and slices of lemon. This makes a delicious cooling drink for hot weather.

LIQUID FOOD

Under this heading such liquids are given as are actual foods.

Milk. Milk is a complete food and a perfect
food for infants, but not a perfect food for adults.
It may be used as
  Whole or skimmed;
  Peptonized; boiled;
  Sterilized; pasteurized;
  Milk with lime water, Vichy or Apollinaris;
  With equal parts of farinaceous liquids;
  Albuminized milk with white of egg;
  Milk with egg yolk, flavored with vanilla, cinnamon,
or nutmeg;
  Milk flavored with coffee, cocoa, or meat broth;
  Milk punch; milk lemonade;
  Kumys; kefir or whey, with lemon juice, as above.

Milk and Cinnamon. Boil in one pint of new milk sufficient
cinnamon to flavor it and sweeten with white sugar.

Egg Preparations. These consist of:
  Albumin water (diluted white of egg), flavored with
fruit juice;
  Egg lemonade; egg orangeade;
  Egg with meat broth;
  Egg with coffee and milk;
  Chocolate eggnog.
  Often the white of egg, dissolved in water or milk,
is given when the yolk cannot be digested because of
the amount of fat which it contains.
  When one is inclined to biliousness, the egg is better
digested if beaten in wine.
  The albuminous or egg drinks are best prepared
cold.

Eggnog. To make eggnog, separate the white and the yolk,
beat the yolk with three-quarters of a tablespoonful of sugar and

a speck of salt until creamy. Add three-quarters of a cup of milk and 1 tablespoonful of brandy. Beat the white until foamy, add to the above mixture, and serve immediately. A little nutmeg may be substituted for the brandy. The eggs and milk should be chilled before using. Eggnog is very nutritious.

Egg Broth. Beat the yolk of 1 egg, add 1 tablespoonful of sugar and a speck of salt. Add 1 cup of hot milk and pour it on gradually. Flavor with nutmeg.

Dried and rolled bread crumbs may be added, or beef, mutton, or chicken broth may be used in place of the milk, and the sugar may be omitted. The whole egg may be used if desired.

This is very delicious made with beef broth, instead of hot milk. Pineapple juice or coffee may be used.

Coffee Eggnog. 1 egg, 1¼ teaspoons of sugar, one-half scant cup of milk or cream, one-half scant cup of coffee.

Egg Malted Milk. Mix 1 tablespoonful of Horlick's Malted Milk with 1 tablespoonful of crushed fruit and 1 egg; beat for five minutes. Strain and add 20 drops of acid phosphate, 1 tablespoonful of crushed ice, and three-quarters cup of ice water. A grating of nutmeg may be used for flavor.

Grape Yolk. Separate the white and the yolk of an egg, beat the yolk, add the sugar, and let the yolk and sugar stand while the white of the egg is thoroughly whipped. Add 2 tablespoonfuls of grape juice to the yolk and pour this on to the beaten white, blending carefully. Have all ingredients chilled before blending and serve cold.

Albuminized Milk. Beat one-half cup of milk and the white of 1 egg with a few grains of salt. Put into a fruit jar, shake thoroughly until blended. Strain into a glass and serve cold.

White Wine Whey. To half a pint of milk boiling add 1 wine-glassful of sherry. Strain through a cheesecloth. Sweeten with powdered sugar to taste. For a child give a tablespoonful every 2 or 3 hours.

Albumin Water. Albumin water is used chiefly for infants in cases of acute stomach and intestinal disorders, in which some nutritious and easily assimilated food is needed. The white of 1 egg is beaten and mixed with a pint of water, which has been boiled and cooled.

Albuminized Grape Juice. Put 2 tablespoonfuls of grape juice into a dainty glass with pure chopped ice. Beat the white of 1 egg, turn into the glass, sprinkle a little sugar over the top, and serve.

Cream of Tartar Water. Dissolve a teaspoonful or a teaspoonful and a half of cream of tartar in a pint of boiling water,
flavor with lemon peel and sugar. Strain and drink when cold.

Farinaceous Beverages. These are all made by
slowly cooking cereals, such as barley, rice, oatmeal,
etc., in a large quantity of boiling water from two to
three hours, straining off the liquid, and seasoning to
taste. They are particularly valuable when only a
small amount of nutriment can be assimilated. Since
the chief ingredient is starch, long cooking is necessary
to make soluble the starch globules, so that it can be
more readily digested. Since these drinks are given
only in case of weak digestion, it is important that
they be taken slowly and held in the mouth until they
are thoroughly mixed with the saliva.

Barley Water (Infant feeding). Mix 1 teaspoonful of barley
flour with 2 tablespoonfuls of cold water, until it is a smooth paste.
Put in the top of a double boiler and add gradually 1 pint of
boiling water. Boil over direct heat five minutes, stirring constantly; then put into a double boiler, over boiling water, and cook
fifteen minutes longer. This is used as a milk diluent for normal
infants and to check diarrhea.

For children or adults use one-half teaspoonful of barley or
rice flour, 1 cup of boiling water, and one-quarter teaspoonful of
salt. Cream or milk and salt may be added for adults, or, lemon
juice and sugar, according to the condition.

Barley water is an astringent and used to check the bowels
when they are too loose.

Barley Water (Bartholow). Wash 2 ounces of pearl barley with
cold water. Then boil it for five minutes in some fresh water and
throw both waters away. Then pour on 2 quarts of boiling water
and boil it down to a quart. Stir and skim occasionally. Flavor
with lemon rind. Add sugar to taste but do not strain unless
the patient requests it.

Rice Water or Mucilage of Rice. Thoroughly wash 1 ounce of
rice with cold water. Then soak for three hours in a quart of

water kept at a tepid heat, stirring from time to time, and after-
wards boil slowly for an hour and strain.   This is useful in dysentery, diarrhea, and irritable states of the alimentary canal.   It
may be sweetened and flavored in the same way as barley water.

Flaxseed Tea.   One-half cupful of flaxseed to 1 quart of boiling
water.   Boil thirty minutes and let stand near the fire to thicken.
Strain, add lemon juice and sugar to taste.

Rice Water.   Wash 2 tablespoonfuls of rice, add 3 cups of cold
water, and soak thirty minutes.   Then heat gradually and cook
one hour until the rice is tender.   Strain through muslin, reheat,
and dilute with boiling water or hot milk to the consistency
desired.   Season with salt; sugar may be added if desired and cinnamon, if allowed, may be cooked with it as a flavor.   One teaspoonful of stoned raisins may be added to the rice, before boiling,
if there is no bowel trouble.

Oatmeal Water.   Mix 1 tablespoonful of oatmeal with 1 tablespoonful of cold water.   Add a speck of salt and stir into it a
quart of boiling water.   Boil for three hours, replenishing the
water as it boils away.   Strain though a fine sieve or cheesecloth, season, and serve cold.   Sufficient water should be added
to keep the drink almost as thin as water.

Toast Water.   Toast thin slices of stale bread in the oven;
break up into crumbs; add 1 cup of boiling water and let it stand
for an hour.   Rub through a fine strainer, season with a little
salt.   Milk, or cream and sugar may be added if desirable.   This
is valuable in cases of fever or extreme nausea.

Sago Soup.   Stew 2 ounces of the best sago in a pint of water
until it is quite tender.   Mix with half a pint of good boiling
cream and the yolks of two fresh eggs.   Put into it 1 quart of
essence of beef.   Mix thoroughly.   The beef essence must be
heated separately and mixed while both mixtures are hot.   This
must be served warm.

Crust Coffee.   Dry crusts of brown bread in the oven until they
are hard and crisp.   Pound or roll them and pour boiling water
over.   Let soak for fifteen minutes, then strain carefully through
a fine sieve.

MEAT JUICES

Meat juice may be prepared in three ways:

(1) Broil quickly, or even scorch, a small piece of

beef. Squeeze out the juice with a lemon squeezer, previously dipped in boiling water. Catch the juice in a hot cup. Season and serve. If desirable to heat it further, place the cup in hot water.

(2) Broil quickly, cut up and put the small pieces into a glass jar. Set the covered jar in a pan of cold water. Heat gradually for an hour, never allowing the water to come to a boil. Strain and press out the clear, red juice, season, and serve. One pound of beef yields 8 tablespoonfuls of juice.'

(3) Grind raw beef and place in a lightly covered jar with 1 gill of cold water to a pound of beef. Stand it on ice overnight and squeeze through a bag. Strain, season, and serve.

Meat Tea. Meat tea is made by using a pound of meat to a pint of water. Grind the meat, place in a jar, and cover with the cold water. Set the jar in an open kettle of water and cook for two hours or more, not allowing the water to boil. Strain by squeezing through a bag, skim off the fat, and season.

Meat Broth. Meat broth is made from meat and bone, with or without vegetables. The proportion is a quart of water to a pound of meat. Cut the meat into small pieces, add the cold water, and simmer until the quantity is reduced one-half. Strain, skim, and season with salt. Chicken, veal, mutton, and beef may be used in this way. It may be seasoned with onions, celery, bay-leaves, cloves, carrots, parsnips, rice, barley, or tapioca. Stale bread crumbs may be added.

Mutton and Chicken Broth. Cut up a chicken or a pound of mutton, because it is free from fat, put into cold water to cover, and let stand on ice two or three hours. Cook over a slow fire until the meat falls from the bone. Strain, cool, skim off the fat, salt to taste, and allow to cool. This may be served hot or cold.

Broth for the Sick. To 1 pound of chopped lean meat of any kind, except pork or veal, add 1 pint of cold water or one pint and a half on ice. Let stand in a covered glass fruit jar for from four to six hours, cook for three hours in a closed jar placed in a kettle of water, strain, cool, skim off the fat, clear with a beaten egg, season to taste. This may be given warm or cold.

Beef Tea and Oatmeal. Two tablespoonfuls of oatmeal and 2 of cold water, mix thoroughly. Add a pint of good beef tea which has been brought to the boiling point. Boil together for five minutes. The oatmeal must have been previously cooked for a long time. It may be taken from that prepared for the morning meal.

Soups. Clear soups are made by cooking raw meat or vegetables, or both together, slowly, for a long time, then straining the liquid. The flavor may be changed by browning the meat or vegetables in butter before adding the water.

Cream soups are made in the proportion of 1 quart of vegetables (such as corn, peas, beans, tomatoes, celery, or asparagus) to 1 pint of water and adding 1 pint of milk. Cook the vegetables thoroughly in water and mash through a colander. To this water and pulp add a cream sauce made in the proportion of 4 tablespoonfuls of flour, 4 tablespoonfuls of butter, and 1 pint of milk, for vegetables poor in starch or protein. Add 2 tablespoonfuls of flour, 2 tablespoonfuls of butter, and a pint of milk for those rich in protein. Season to taste.

Tomato acid should be counteracted by the addition of one-eighth tablespoonful of soda before the milk is added.

Potato soup may be flavored with onion or celery, or both.

SEMI-SOLID FOODS

The following lists of foods are given for ready reference:[1]

Jellies.

    (a) Meat jellies and gelatin; veal, beef, chicken, mutton.
    (b) Starch jellies, flavored with fruit; cornstarch, arrowroot, sago, tapioca.
    (c) Fruit jellies and gelatin.

[1] *Nutrition and Dietetics*, by Dr. W. S. Hall, D. Appleton & Co., New York.

Custards.
    (a) Junkets of milk, or milk and egg (rennet curdled),
        flavored with nutmeg, etc.
    (b) Egg, milk custard, boiled or baked.
    (c) Cornstarch, tapioca, boiled custard.
    (d) Frozen custard (New York ice cream.)

Gruels. (Farinaceous.)
    (a) Milk gruels.
    (b) Water gruels.

Jellies.—Meat Jellies are made in two ways:

(1) Cook soup meat (containing gristle and bone) slowly for a long time in just enough water to cover. Strain and set the liquid away in a mold to cool and set. If desired, bits of shredded meat may be added to the liquid before molding.

(2) Use meat broth and gelatin in the proportion of 1 tablespoon gelatin to three-quarters of a cup of hot broth. Pour into mold and set on ice.

Starch Jellies. Starch jellies are made by cooking in a pint of fruit juice or water until clear, 2 tablespoonfuls of tapioca, arrowroot, sago, cornstarch, or flour. Sweeten to taste.

If water is used, fresh fruit may be used either in the jelly or in a sauce poured over the jelly.

Fruit Jellies. These are made:

(1) Of fruit juice and sugar in equal quantities, cooked until it will set when cooled;

(2) Of fruit juice and gelatin in the proportion of 1 tablespoon of gelatin to three-fourths of a cup of fruit juice, or one-half box gelatin to 1½ pints of juice. Sugar to taste. Made tea or coffee, or cocoa or lemonade may be used in the same proportion.

Custards. These are made with (1) milk, (2) milk and eggs, (3) milk, egg, and some farinaceous substances as rice, cornstarch, tapioca. In the first the coagulum is produced by the addition of rennet, in the other two by the application of heat.

Plain Junket. Dissolve in a cup of lukewarm milk (never warmer), a tablespoon of sugar or caramel syrup. Add a quarter of a junket tablet, previously dissolved in a tablespoon of cold water. Stir a few times, add vanilla, nuts, or nutmeg if desired. Pour into a cup and set aside to cool and solidify. This may be served plain or with whipped cream, or boiled custard.

Egg-Milk Custard. When eggs are used for thickening, not less than four eggs should be used to a quart of milk (more eggs make it richer).

Snowballs. Heat 1 pint of milk with sugar to taste. Beat the whites of 3 eggs stiff, then beat in 1½ tablespoonfuls of powdered sugar. Drop by spoonfuls into the hot milk, turn in three minutes, and take out. Beat yolks of the eggs, pour the hot milk over them, and allow to thicken. Do not boil. Arrange snowballs in dish and pour custard over. Serve cool.

Boiled Custard. One pint of milk, 2 eggs, one-half cup of sugar, one-half saltspoon of salt. Scald the milk, add the salt and sugar, and stir until dissolved. Beat the eggs very thick and smooth. Pour the boiling milk on the eggs slowly, stirring all the time. Pour the mixture into a double boiler, set over the fire, and stir for ten minutes. Add flavoring. As soon as a thickening of the mixture is noticed remove from the fire, pour into a dish, and set away to cool. This custard makes *cup custard*, the sauce for such puddings as *snow pudding*, and when decorated with spoonfuls of beaten egg-white, makes *floating island*.

Baked Custard. Proceed as in boiled custard, but instead of pouring into a double boiler pour into a baking dish. Set the dish in a pan of water, place in the oven, and bake until the mixture is set in the middle.

Farinaceous Custards. Make like boiled custard, using one less egg and adding one-quarter cup of farina, tapioca, cornstarch, arrowroot, or cooked rice to the hot milk and egg.

Sago should be soaked overnight before using.

Tapioca should be soaked one hour before using.

Coffee Custard. Scald one tablespoon of ground coffee in milk and strain before proceeding as for boiled custard.

Chocolate Custard. Add one square of grated chocolate to the milk.

Caramel Custard. Melt the dry sugar until golden brown, add the hot milk, and when dissolved proceed as before. Bake.

Milk for Puddings or Stewed Fruit (Ringer). Boil a small piece of lemon rind and 2 cloves in a pint of milk. Mix half a teaspoon-full of arrowroot in a little cold milk and add it to the boiled milk. Stir until about the consistency of cream. Beat up the yolks of 3 eggs in a little milk. Beat into the hot milk taken off the fire and as it cools add the eggs and a tablespoonful of orange flower water, stirring it constantly until quite cool. Keep in a very cool place until required for use.

Bread Jelly. Pour boiling water on stale bread and allow it to soak until soft. Pour off the water, add fresh water to cover, and boil until stiff and until it becomes jelly-like when it cools. It may be eaten with milk or cream.

SOLID FOODS

(Suitable for Invalids)

Toasts.
    (a) Cream toast.
    (b) Milk toast.
    (c) Water toast.

Creams.
    (a) Plain.
    (b) Whipped.
    (c) Ice cream.

Oils.
    (a) Plain olive, cotton seed, or nut.
    (b) Butter.
    (c) Emulsion, as mayonnaise.
    (d) Cod-liver oil, plain or emulsified.

Cereals.
    (a) Porridges and mushes—Oatmeal, corn meal, wheat, rice, etc.
    (b) Dry preparations—Shredded wheat biscuit, corn flakes, puffed rice, puffed wheat, triscuit.

Breads.
    (a) Plain—White, Graham, nutri-meal, whole wheat, brown, rye, etc.
    (b) Toasts—Dry, buttered, zwieback.
    (c) Crackers—Soda, Graham, oatmeal, Boston butter, milk.
    (d) Biscuits—Yeast biscuits (twenty-four hours old), baking-powder biscuit, beaten biscuit.

Egg Preparations.
> (a) Boiled, poached, scrambled, baked.
> (b) Omelets.
> (c) Souffles of meat and of potatoes.

Meats.
> (a) Beef or mutton—Broiled or roasted.
> (b) Chicken, turkey, or game—Broiled or roasted.
> (c) Fish—Broiled, boiled, or baked.
> (d) Oysters—Canned, stewed, etc.
> (e) Clams—Chowder, broiled, or baked.

Vegetables.
> (a) Potatoes—Baked, boiled, creamed, or escalloped.
> (b) Sweet potatoes, baked or boiled.
> (d) Lima beans, plain or creamed; string beans, plain or creamed; cauliflower, plain or creamed; carrots; parsnips.
> (c) Green peas, plain or creamed.
> (d) Lima beans, plain or creamed; string beans, plain or creamed; cauliflower, plain or creamed; carrots; parsnips.

Fruits.
> (a) Fresh—Oranges, grapes, melons, etc.
> (b) Stewed—Apples, plums, apricots, pears, berries, etc.
> (c) Baked—Apples, bananas, pears.
> (d) Canned—Peaches, apricots, plums, pears, etc.
> (e) Preserved—Peaches, plums, quinces, etc.

Gruels. Gruels are a mixture of grain or flour with either milk or water. They require long cooking and may be flavored with sugar, nutmeg, cinnamon, or almond.

Take the meal or flour (oatmeal, 2 tablespoons, or corn meal, 1 tablespoon, or arrowroot, 1¼ tablespoons). Sift it slowly into 1½ cups boiling water, simmer for an hour or two. Strain off the liquid; add to it 1 teaspoon of sugar, season with salt, and add 1 cup of warm milk.

Water Gruel. If water gruel is desired, let the last cup of liquid added be water instead of milk.

Cream Gruel.   A cream gruel may be made by using rich cream instead of milk or water.

Barley Gruel.   Barley gruel (usually a water gruel) is prepared as follows: Moisten 4 tablespoons of barley flour in a little cold water and add it slowly to the boiling water.   Stir and boil for twenty minutes.

Toasts.—Cream Toast.   Toast the bread slowly until brown on both sides.   Butter and pour over each slice enough warm cream to moisten (the cream may be thickened slightly and the butter may be omitted).

Milk Toast.   One tablespoon of cornstarch or flour; one cup of milk, salt to taste, and boil.   Butter the toast and pour over it the above white sauce.

Water Toast.   Pour over plain or buttered toast enough boiling water to thoroughly moisten it.

Souffles of Fruit, etc.   The distinguished feature of a souffle is a pastry or pulpy foundation mixture, and the addition of stiffly beaten egg-white. A souffle may or may not be baked.

Plain Souffle.   Two tablespoons flour; 1 cup of liquid (water, milk, or fruit juice); 3 or 4 eggs; sugar to suit the fruit.   If thick fruit pulp is used, omit the thickening.   Beat the egg-yolks until thick.   Add sugar gradually and continue beating.   Add the fruit (if lemon juice add some rind also).   Fold in the well-beaten whites.   Bake in a buttered dish (set in a pan of hot water) for thirty-five or forty minutes in a slow oven.

Fresh Fruit Souffle.   Reduce the fruit to a pulp.   Strawberries, peaches, prunes, apples, bananas, etc., may be used.   Sweeten the pulp.   Beat the egg-white to a stiff froth, add the fruit pulp slowly.   Chill and serve with whipped cream or soft custard.

Chocolate Souffle.   Two tablespoons flour; 2 tablespoons butter; three-quarters cup of milk; one-third cup of sugar; 2 tablespoons hot water.   Melt the butter, add the flour, and stir well.   Pour the milk in gradually and cook until well boiled.   Add the melted chocolate, to which the sugar and hot water have been added.

Beat in the yolks and fold in the whites of the eggs. Bake twenty-five minutes.

Farina Souffle. Cook the farina (4 tablespoons) in a pint of boiling water. Stir this with the egg-yolks, add sugar or salt, and later fold in the egg-whites, flavor, and set away to cool.

CHAPTER XII

INFANT FEEDING

ONE of the fundamental problems of to-day, as it was of yesterday and will be of to-morrow, is the correct feeding of infants and children.

Every civilized country faces the same problem, largely because the artificial feeding of infants has become so prevalent.

Unfortunately, many women who must labor outside of the home must resort partially, if not entirely, to artificial feeding of their infants. Usually on account of the inconvenience of breast feeding and the strain on the mother, the infant is given artificial food, often improperly prepared. Although infant mortality is high among the poorer classes, it is marvelous that so many of these infants survive.

It is an encouraging fact, however, that women among the well-to-do and educated classes are appreciating the importance of breast feeding and that the number of these who are not only willing but anxious to nurse their infants is increasing.

The mother should be firm in her decision to nurse her child and be encouraged to persevere in efforts to secure the proper development of the breasts before the birth of the child, that the quantity as well as the quality of the milk may be adequate.

The fact that nearly one-fourth of the civilized race dies during the first year of life is astounding. This mortality is due directly or indirectly to nutritional disturbances that could in a great measure be prevented if the babies were properly nursed at the breast or if the artificial feeding was carefully regulated.

Of six hundred and forty-one infants under observation by Dublin, in Fall River, Mass., five hundred and sixty-five were breast-fed and seventy-six bottle-fed. After the first week there were one hundred and six deaths. In seventy-four of these the infants were breast-fed, and in thirty-two, bottled-fed; nearly one-half of the bottle-fed babies died and only 10 per cent. of the breast-fed babies. The breast-fed child, therefore, has five chances to live where the bottle-fed child has one.

One fundamental principle on which all of the leading specialists in the study of the baby agree, is that the milk of the healthy mother is the only ideal baby food. Every mother should be made to realize the importance of nursing her baby for at least nine or ten months, unless circumstances beyond control make it impossible or inadvisable.

Proper care of the breasts and of the general health during the expectant period will usually secure a sufficient flow of milk for the child's needs.

The mental attitude of the mother has much to do with the secretion of milk; therefore she should cultivate the habit of kindly, cheerful, healthful thoughts. She should keep her circulation and vitality up to par.

She should take regular exercise and be out in the fresh air daily.

During the first two or three days the child receives little nourishment from the breast, simply a few ounces daily of a yellowish substance known as colostrum, which is supposed to have a laxative effect on its bowels.

It is, however, usual to put the child to the breast at regular intervals of about four hours after the first day, to stimulate the milk secretion, which should be quite free on the third day; it, however, may be slow in coming for a day to two longer.

A teaspoonful or two of warm boiled water, or of a five per cent. solution of milk-sugar may be given every few hours, in fact it is considered advisable by some physicians, in order to lessen somewhat the loss in weight which takes place during the first week.

If the free flow of milk is delayed beyond forty-eight hours, some nourishment must be given. A little modified cow's milk is best. The preparation of this will be taken up under Artificial Feeding.

The mother should not permit herself to become easily discouraged about her ability to nurse her child, for even though the supply at first seems very deficient and it is necessary to give the baby other nourishment, it should be put to the breast at regular intervals, as the sucking by the child stimulates the secretion of milk. The flow of milk often increases when the mother becomes more active.

When the milk flows freely, the contents of one breast is sufficient for one nursing, and the breasts should be used alternately, that is one breast at one feeding and the other at the next.

Nursing should not last longer than from ten to twenty minutes. Too rapid nursing is apt to cause vomiting. If it is necessary to check the flow of milk somewhat, it can be done by pressing the breast slightly between the fingers.

There is a warmth, a purity, and a vitality to the mother's milk that is impossible to secure in any artificial food no matter how carefully and skilfully prepared. It is also germ-free.

Some women seem unable to nurse their babies for more than two or three months and it is sometimes thought that it is not worth while for a woman to nurse her baby unless she can do so for a considerable time. This, however, is a great mistake, because there is no time in the baby's life when it is more important for it to have breast milk than in the beginning. This is the time when the baby's digestion is most easily disturbed and most difficult to correct. Every day or week that a baby gets breast milk gives it a better start.

It has been thought that it is dangerous to use both breast and artificial feeding. This idea is erroneous. The artificial food cannot make the breast milk hard to digest, while the breast feeding seems to make the artificial food digest more readily. This may be due in part to the ferments which the breast milk contains, but more probably is due to the fact that the baby is able to utilize the proteins of human milk to build tissue when it cannot so readily utilize the proteins of the artificial food.

Wet nursing is resorted to less frequently now than in the past on account of better methods for artificial feeding. **Wet Nursing**

If the mother is unable to nurse the child herself and the conditions are ideal, that is the wet nurse a healthy, happy woman with a thriving baby of her own, and very particular in the care of her person, this is better than artificial feeding.

Contra-Indications to Nursing Total absence of milk, after earnest efforts to stimulate its secretion necessitates artificial feeding.

If the mother has chorea, epilepsy, or tuberculosis in any form, it is best to resort to artificial feeding; also if the mother has syphilis and the baby is free from it. In these conditions the child must often be taken from the mother to avoid infection.

If the mother has had serious complications in pregnancy or parturition, the physician must decide on the advisability of natural or artificial feeding.

In case of nephritis, except perhaps in a very mild form, the milk is toxic and therefore nursing from the breast should be prohibited.

Sometimes in acute contagious disease it is safer to nurse the baby than to subject it to the dangers of artificial food. However, when the mother's temperature exceeds 101 or 102 degrees, the milk will probably possess toxic qualities and disagree with the infant.

Anatomy and Physiology of the Infant Every nursing mother should acquaint herself with the process of the infant's digestion, as many of the infantile difficulties are caused by overfeeding or underfeeding, due to ignorance on this subject.

The alimentary tract of the new-born infant differs in many ways from that of the adult.

As compared with other mammals, the human infant is the most helpless and undeveloped and therefore the most delicate and easily affected. It is practically dependent on its mother for nourishment which will completely supply its needs.

The capacity of the stomach, after careful study,

has been placed at from 1 to 2 ounces at birth, 2 to 3 ounces at the end of the first month, 6 ounces at the 6th month, and from 9 to 10 ounces at the end of the first year. This is simply an average guide, as stomachs vary somewhat in size. Quantities somewhat larger than the foregoing are sometimes fed, but some of the food has passed beyond the pylorus before the last of it is taken. Digestion begins as soon as the food enters the stomach.

The secretion of bile begins within 12 hours after birth, increases rapidly, and is fully established within a week or ten days.

The pancreatic ferments which digest starches and sugar are present in the new-born, although scanty; the sucking movements of the child when nursing exercise the salivary glands so that saliva is secreted; but starch digestion is not completed in the mouth, hence starch and a greater proportion of sugar than is in the mother's milk are difficult for the infant to digest.

The intestines, when compared with the length of the body, are relatively long in infants, but the muscular coat is comparatively weak; digestion is therefore relatively slow and more subject to derangement by substances that influence peristalsis.

The fact that infants vomit with comparatively little effort, the food overflowing from an overloaded stomach, is due to the relatively feeble closure of the cardiac orifice.

The stomach contents are kept germ-free by the secretion of hydrochloric acid and the upper intestine is nearly free from bacteria in breast-fed infants, because of the antibacterial nature of the intestinal secretion. In some digestive disturbances this safeguard fails and bacteria develop rapidly.

Intestinal Disturbances
Intestinal disturbance in the breast-fed infant is most often caused by overfeeding, the infant often nursing too frequently, thereby emptying the breasts and securing a high fat ratio. Frequent nursing does not give the stomach time to empty and thus digestive disturbances are apt to occur. Therefore, as a means of relieving intestinal trouble in the infant, nursing at regular intervals and not too frequently, is of much importance.

When digestive disturbance has occurred it is best to stop nursing for twenty-four hours, giving the infant weak barley gruel sweetened with saccharin. At the end of twenty-four hours let the infant nurse at the breast for from three to five minutes, this being preceded by a small drink of water.

As the bowel condition improves, the time at the breast may be gradually lengthened.

The mother should watch her diet to avoid too much rich food, and foods that seem difficult to digest, as certain articles of food in the mother's diet often causes gastric disturbances in the infant.

She should also carefully watch her thoughts, keeping them well poised and upon kindness, love, and peace. Worry or unkind thoughts will affect the mother's milk and disturb the child's digestion very quickly.

Fits of temper in the child also disturb its digestion.

Times of Feeding
Regular nursing habits should be insisted on, as indigestion, colic, and diarrhea often result from irregular nursing.

Some authorities discourage night feeding as unnecessary with a normal baby, but most physicians agree that the child should be aroused during the day in order not to miss a feeding, as it will fall asleep again directly after nursing and will soon get into the habit of awakening at feeding time.

The following table from Holt may be used as a guide in breast-feeding:

Age	Number in twenty-four hours	Intervals during the day hours	Night nursing between 9 P.M. and 7 A.M.
1st day.............	4	6	1
2d day.............	6	4	1
3d to 28th day......	10	2	2
4th to 13th week....	8	2½	1
3d to 5th month....	7	3	1
5th to 12th month..	6	3	0

There may be some slight deviations from this if the child is ill and small for its age. It is a good general rule to feed the child according to the age with which its weight corresponds.

There can be no regular rule followed for all. Some authorities hold that fifteen- to twenty-minute feedings at four-hour intervals during the day, with one feeding at night, are sufficient, but it depends on the child. Some babies' stomachs are smaller than others, and some do not nurse regularly, but play and are inattentive to the nursing. In either event the child will not get sufficient nourishment at four-hour intervals. The intelligent mother can determine what is best.

In breast-feeding, as well as in most of the formulæ for bottle-feeding, there is an **Water** allowance for an amount of fluid that, under ordinary circumstances, satisfies the baby's requirements.

Additional water is often necessary, especially during the hot weather when the body heat is regulated through evaporation from the skin. The most effective means of promoting perspiration is the giving of water. This, however, should not be done to excess. Eight ounces for a 10-pound baby, given in divided doses during the day, will be sufficient.

It is best to give the water when the stomach is nearly or quite empty. It should be boiled and cooled and should be given by the bottle as the child will then take at intervals all that its thirst requires, and the danger of choking as a result of too hasty swallowing is avoided.

Normal Development in the Breast-Fed The growth and general condition of the child will, of course, be influenced by the quality and quantity of the milk. The birth weight of 7 to 7½ pounds is usually doubled by the end of the fifth month and trebled by the end of the year. The average gain is from 5 to 8 ounces a week during the first few months and from 2 to 4 ounces a week the last few months of the year.

If the mother's milk is deficient in any way, the child becomes fretful and loses weight, or the weight remains stationary. In such cases the physician usually examines the milk to determine its quality and advises some means of improving it, or in some way adding to the baby's food the element in which the mother's milk is lacking.

The physical condition of the mother often affects the baby's nourishment, and besides resorting, temporarily, to means for improving the quality of the milk, she should build up her general vitality through regular exercise for the spine and the vital organs, deep breathing of fresh air, and regular rest.

While a scanty food supply will diminish the flow of milk, overloading the stomach at meal time and taking quantities of rich food between meals, as so many nursing mothers, think is necessary, usually does little to increase the quantity or improve the quality of the milk, but often results in an accumulation of superfluous flesh and disturbed digestion, which quickly affects the child.

Sometimes a more restricted diet together with specially directed exercises to relieve any digestive disturbance and correct constipation, and relaxing exercises for the nerves, will do more than anything else to improve the quality of the milk.

Mothers should particularly avoid becoming overtired.

When the milk is good, but the quantity deficient, massage of the breasts three or four times a day for five or ten minutes will increase the supply. One effective means of increasing the secretion of the mammary glands is the mechanical stimulus of suction. If a robust baby can be put to the breast for a time it may develop an ample flow of milk for a puny infant whose powers of suction are feeble.

A good malt extract with meals sometimes tends to increase the flow of milk. When the quality and quantity of the milk are deficient, the physician usually advises a very nourishing diet and a tonic. This nourishment does not of necessity require an excessive amount of liquid.

When the quantity is sufficient, but the quality poor, it is usually necessary to wean the baby, if it is several months old, although mother's milk, even if below standard in quality, is better for the infant than cow's milk, at least during the first few months.

Nervousness, sleeplessness, worry, and grief have a decided effect on the milk supply and on the baby. Nervous mothers are apt to have an abundance of milk one day and little the next day; frequently the milk will disappear suddenly.

Weaning   When it is possible, the baby should be weaned gradually. Although there is no set time for weaning, it is not advisable to feed the child exclusively from the breast after the eighth or tenth month. Bunge holds that human milk contains too little iron at this period and the babies are apt to become pale and undernourished.

When additional feeding is decided on, the physician should prescribe the preparation. A bottle a day should be substituted for the breast feeding at first and, gradually, additional bottle feedings, until, after about a month the breast is entirely withdrawn.

After the eighth month and until the age of twelve months, as a general rule, cow's milk should be diluted and sweetened by mixing eight ounces of barley water and thirty-two ounces of milk, adding an ounce of cane-sugar or milk-sugar, and dividing the whole into five 8-ounce portions.

Additional food may be given to the healthy child after the eighth or ninth month. Orange juice or other fruit juice one or twice a day should be given about an hour before feeding. A teaspoonful may be given at first and the amount gradually increased to about two tablespoonfuls a day.

Orange juice is a specific in conditions of scurvy

resulting from improper feeding. The child usually improves rapidly after it begins to take the juice.

Beef juice, meat broths, or strained vegetable soup may be given in increasing amounts up to 5 or 6 ounces daily.

Zwieback and whole wheat or Graham crackers are permissible in small amounts after the ninth month. After nine months the healthy baby should also have a soft-boiled egg occasionally, also baked apple and well-cooked, mashed spinach or carrots.

Food should be given only at regular intervals and nothing but water between feedings.

Starch-digesting ferments are present at birth in sufficient amounts to digest the sugar in milk, but they do not develop sufficiently to digest starches until about the twelfth month, so white bread, crackers made from white flour, potatoes, rice, etc., should not be given the child under a year.

When artificial feeding is necessary, the physician must decide what modification is best for the baby. One can only determine by experimenting upon the actual percentages of fat, proteins, and sugar which each baby needs, following, in general, the proportions contained in mother's milk, because while many babies thrive on a food of this composition, some do not. The formulæ given are simply a guide, as the proportions may need to be changed, or may need to be made weaker in some cases and stronger in others. **Artificial Feeding**

The composition of human milk, however, is a guide to the infant's digestive ability. This must be determined by a careful study of the *individual baby* as every baby is a problem by itself.

As previously mentioned, no artificial food is the same as human milk, although it may contain the same proportions of the different elements, and it is often difficult, especially during the first few months, to prepare a combination on which the child will thrive.

Cow's milk, properly prepared, is the nearest available substitute for human milk. It must be modified, as the digestion of the calf at birth is equal to that of an infant at eight or nine months.

Farmers have in recent years become more particular about the care of their cows and cleanliness in milking because the educational campaign with regard to the danger to human life from tuberculous animals has caused a greater public demand for good, clean milk.

Many infectious diseases are conveyed by milk, and impure milk is a large cause of the extraordinarily high mortality of early infancy. With the improvement of the milk supply, the decline in the infant death-rate has been wondrously gratifying.

Manufacturers have taken advantage of the fact that the public has become a little afraid of cow's milk and have extensively advertised their prepared foods, claiming them to be the best substitute for mother's milk. However, experiments have proven that these statements for the most part are misleading, the composition of the foods not being suited to the actual requirements of the infant. Some prominent physicians think that infant mortality has been increasing since prepared foods have been used so extensively.

One leading authority states that "clean, fresh cow's milk, properly modified, is the best substitute available. It is to be preferred to any prepared food, no matter how sweeping may be the manufacturers' claim for it."

The most striking thing about the prepared foods is their tremendous excess of carbohydrates, either cane-sugar or sugar derived from starch by the process of malting. Condensed milk, in particular, contains much too large a percentage of cane-sugar for the child.

Another authority states:

An excess of sugar is likely to damage the organism by the production of poisonous substances in the body. This is particularly true in those infants who are already suffering from indigestion. An excess of sugar in such a baby is likely to render him severely and dangerously sick and result in catastrophe.

The study of the bacteriology of the alimentary tract of the new-born infant **Bacteriology** reveals a most interesting fact and explains why artificial feeding is often so difficult and dangerous.

In the intestinal canal at all times many varieties of vegetable organisms (bacteria) are present. These are called floral organisms. Some of these aid digestion while some others increase disturbance in the intestines, particularly if in excess, or if digestive derangements occur.

The flora which predominate are those peculiar to the infant which is properly digesting human milk. This accounts for the uniform action of the bowels in breast-fed infants. As soon as the child gets milk from the breast, the intestinal flora assume this definite form.

When cow's milk or any other food is given, the intestinal flora change. When the change is made too suddenly, these new flora which live on the digested products of human milk gradually disappear and the

action of the new flora often causes intestinal derangements which the infant is not strong enough to overcome.

Composition of Human Milk If artificial feeding must be resorted to, the composition should resemble mother's milk as nearly as possible. It is impossible to duplicate it exactly and even though the elements and the proportion of them are the same, the bacterial flora will be different and consequently the effect also.

If the breasts are emptied regularly, human milk varies little in composition after the first few weeks. According to Holt there is an average in mother's milk of

Fat	4%
Sugar	7%
Protein	1.5%
Salt	0.2%
Water	87.3%

Adaptation of Cow's Milk When the baby has been fed at the breast for several months, pure cow's milk some-times agrees very well, if overfeeding is avoided.

The amount of milk taken every twenty-four hours by a healthy infant is usually about 1¼ ounces to the pound of the baby's weight.

A normal infant of twelve pounds would be taking between twelve and eighteen ounces of milk in its twenty-four hour mixture.

Budin recommends one-tenth of the body-weight daily of milk and reports excellent results in infants after the fifth or sixth month, weighing from thirteen to fifteen pounds.

Most infants under the age of nine months are more or less incapable of digesting cow's milk undiluted. If artificial food is resorted to from the start, practically all physicians agree that the milk should be diluted or otherwise modified during the first few months at least.

Milk diluted with water is often given, one part of milk to two parts of water. This reduces the protein to about the amount found in breast milk.

It is necessary to keep up the proportion of protein, as this alone contains the important food element, nitrogen. From one-half to three-fourths of an ounce of milk-sugar is added to the twenty-four hours' supply of food to approximate the seven per cent. found in breast milk.

The proportion of milk and milk-sugar is gradually increased and the water decreased, so that at the end of the first or second month the baby gets equal parts of milk and water and about an ounce more of milk-sugar. This process is continued until, near the end of the first year, the child is on whole milk. The sugar is lessened as the water is omitted.

If, after a few months, it is desired to give a baby starch in its food, cereal waters made of barley, rice, wheat, or oatmeal may be used in place of plain water.

As cow's milk leaves the stomach more slowly than mother's milk, longer intervals between feeding seem advisable. When the breast-fed infant receives nourishment every two and one-half to three hours, an infant given a cow's-milk preparation would be fed every three and one-half or four hours.

The most important thing is to prevent both overfeeding and underfeeding as these are often the greatest factors in producing infantile disturbances. A too rapid gain in weight, (from 8 to 12 ounces a week), which often occurs in artificially fed infants, is not a good sign.

Milk prepared according to the formula desired by the physician can now be secured from milk laboratories in all of our larger cities. However, the milk is apt to spoil in transit, and to secure its freshness when one is not in or near a large city, it is best to prepare it at home. Any intelligent mother or nurse can do this very satisfactorily if the physician gives definite instructions.

Its careful preparation is quite as important as the correct formula.

Mineral (calcium) and protein are bone and other tissue builders, and it is a significant fact that cow's milk contains about twice as much protein and a little more than twice as much of the mineral as mother's milk, indicating that the growth of the human infant is to be slow. The calf requires about four years for full growth and the human being twenty-one years. Both human and cow's milk, however, contain an equal amount of fat, the heat-producing element, as Nature intended that the infant should be warm and active.

It seems almost impossible to get milk from the cow as clean and free from bacteria as it should be and therefore sterilization and pasteurization are resorted to almost universally. Various substances such as formaldehyd, boric acid, and salicylic acid are used by dealers to preserve the milk. These all have a deleterious effect on the child. Therefore the safety of the child demands that the mother choose a reliable dairy. The milk may be analyzed occasionally to make sure of its purity.

A very popular milk preparation and one frequently prescribed by physicians is the top-milk method as originated by Dr. Holt. **Top-Milk**

Top-milk is that at the top of milk bottles in which milk has been allowed to stand for five or six hours.

The cream at the top contains the most fat. For instance, in a quart of milk that has been permitted to stand, the

Upper	4 ounces	contain	20 per cent. of fat.			
"	6 "	"	16 "	"	"	"
"	8 "	"	12 "	"	"	"
"	10 "	"	11 "	"	"	"
"	12 "	"	9 "	"	"	"
"	14 "	"	8 "	"	"	"
"	16 "	"	7 "	"	"	"
"	20 "	"	6 "	"	"	"
"	24 "	"	5 "	"	"	"

To remove the top-milk, the first ounce is taken out with a spoon and the remainder with a Chapin milk dipper which contains one ounce.

The following formula is considered a good top-milk mixture, although it is not supposed to meet the needs of all infants and would therefore have to be modified in some cases and made stronger in others.

TOP-MILK MIXTURE

Top-milk (upper 8 ounces)...........2½ ozs.;
Bottom-milk.......................1 oz.;
Limewater.........................½ oz.;
Milk-sugar........................1 measure (¼ oz.);
Water, sufficient to make............8 ozs.

The sugar is dissolved by boiling it in the quantity of water to be used for the mixture. If not perfectly clear, it is strained through cheesecloth.

The one thing to be particularly guarded against is overloading the stomach with rich food. On account of the high percentage of fat, digestive disturbances often occur when top-milk is used. Some infants can dispose of an abundance of fat from the beginning and most of them can after six or nine months, but many infants have difficulty in digesting fat. The condition called "fat rickets" may exist, though the child may seem to thrive and increase in weight. Its flesh, however, is not hard and firm as it should be in health.

The cream from Guernsey and Jersey cows is usually too rich for infants and therefore the best milk for the baby is that from Holstein or grade cows. The mixed milk from various cows is usually best.

The physician can determine from the stools if the fat ratio is too high, in which case it is best to use top-milk lower in percentage of fat, and lengthen the feeding intervals to four hours.

Certified Milk If the additional expense of certified milk can be met, it is advisable to use it in preparing the baby's food, as it is reasonably constant in its composition and is prepared under the most hygienic conditions, in accordance with the requirements of the American Association of Medical Milk Commissions.

All utensils used in preparing the baby's milk must be absolutely clean. Bacteria develop very quickly in milk and, therefore, the bottles, nipples, etc., should be kept as germ-free as possible by being boiled daily, and the nipples, when not in use, should be kept in a solution of boracic acid (one-fourth ounce boracic acid to one-half pint of water).

The artificially fed baby does not usually thrive as

well as the breast-fed infant. It does not gain in weight as fast and the teeth are slower in coming. The general condition of the baby, and a steady, even if slow gain in weight, will indicate whether the food is agreeing.

Every baby, however, is a law unto itself and it sometimes requires considerable study to determine what is the best food. Even with the utmost care a cow's-milk preparation cannot be made identical with mother's milk and sometimes an entirely different mixture must be resorted to.

However, no mother should attempt to experiment on her baby or permit herself to be misled by the advertisements of so-called Baby Foods. It is only when these are used in the right proportion and in combination with other ingredients that they can be suited to the requirements of the infant.

Malt used in place of milk-sugar or cane-sugar will greatly assist the absorption of fat and decrease the tendency to fermentation and colic. It is being extensively used in milk modifications.

Milk Modifications

It is best to use the dextrin-maltose preparations that do not contain sodium chlorid, as it is rarely advisable to add this salt to the infant's food.

Some physicians have been securing very satisfactory results with a preparation containing whey. Whey is a thin, watery fluid, looking very much like skimmed milk; its caloric value is about 300 per quart, 9 per ounce, barely one-half that of whole milk. It is therefore adapted only to temporary feeding, while its low fat content is of great value in cases of fat dyspepsia.

To secure the whey, 5 grams (1 teaspoonful) of rennet should be used to each quart of milk. The mixture must be kept at a temperature of about 100 F. until it separates into a liquid and a solid portion. It is then strained through cheesecloth. Practically all the casein is left on the cloth, the fluid being the whey. The curd should be broken up before straining, in order to obtain, as nearly as possible, the casein. However, about two-thirds of the milk fats remain in the curd. The whey, besides the whey proteins, thus contains only about one-third of the fats, but nearly all of the milk-sugar and salts. The whey still contains the rennet and, to destroy this, the whey must be heated to at least 140 F. for thirty minutes.

The average composition of whey according to Wachenheim is as follows:

Proteins................	0.8	per cent.
Fats....................	1.0	" "
Milk-sugar.............	4.5	" "
Salts..................	0.7	" "
Water.................	93.0	" "

Sometimes sugar is the primary cause of intestinal fermentation, due to the concentration of the whey and the relative proportions of casein and sugar in the mixture.

According to Finkelstein and Meyer, to prepare a food which will combat intestinal fermentation there must be:

A diminution in the quantity of milk-sugar, a diminution of the salts through dilution of the whey, and an increase in the casein, with varying, and, under certain circumstances, not inconsiderable amounts of fat. After improvement has begun, an easily assimilable and consequently little fermentable carbohydrate should be added.

They developed a food to meet these requirements to which they gave the name of "*Eiweissmilch.*" This food is prepared as follows:

Heat one quart of whole milk to 100 F.; add four teaspoonfuls of essence of pepsin, and stir. Let the mixture stand at 100 F. until the curd has formed, then strain. Press the mass of curd through a rather fine sieve two or three times by the means of a wooden mallet or spoon. Add one pint of water to the curd during this process. The mixture should now look like milk and the precipitate must be very finely divided. Add one pint of buttermilk to this mixture.

Finkelstein and Meyer used buttermilk in the preparation of this food:

(1) Because of the small amount of milk-sugar which it contains;

(2) To obtain the good effects of the lactic acid;

(3) Because buttermilk can be kept for a longer time.

The composition of this food is:

Fat.....................	2.5%
Sugar..................	1.5%
Protein................	3.0%
Salts..................	0.5%

One quart of this milk contains about 360 calories.

They call attention to the low caloric value of this food and to the necessity of increasing it as soon as possible by the addition of dextrin-maltose mixtures.

They claim that it is worthy of employment in all the disturbances of nutrition in infants, which are accompanied by diarrhea, of no matter what kind. The use of this food has been extended by others to all sorts of conditions including the feeding of healthy infants and the newly born, and good results are claimed for it.

To use a food low in sugar and salts and high in protein in the fermentative conditions caused by sugar, is rational. In these conditions the substitution of the dextrin-maltose mixtures for lactose is also good.

Not all disturbances of nutrition accompanied by diarrhea, however, are due to the same cause and should not be treated in the same way. No method of feeding can be applicable to both the sick and the well, nor can all babies be given the same food without regard to their individual digestive ability.

The main principles of this method of treating intestinal fermentative conditions may be used and, at the same time, the disadvantages of a routine food may be avoided, by applying the modification of milk by the percentage method as given by Moise and Talbot.

Sterilizing and Pasteurizing To sterilize the milk it should be heated to 212 F., that temperature being maintained for ten minutes or longer.

Many physicians consider pasteurization the better process. In this the milk is heated to from 150 to 165 F. and kept at that temperature for from twenty to thirty minutes. Boiling produces chemical changes, such as converting the milk-sugar into caramel, etc., while pasteurizing does not.

After pasteurization or sterilization, the milk should be quickly cooled to a temperature of 40 F. or lower and kept, until used, in bottles corked with non-absorbent cotton.

Sterilized or pasteurized milk does not keep as well as raw milk probably on account of the change in the ferments which destroy bacteria; therefore the baby's milk should be pasteurized fresh every day.

Freeman's pasteurizer is a very satisfactory and simple device. It consists of a metal pail into which is fitted a rack with a separate cylinder for each bottle. This holds just enough cold water to surround the bottle and keep it from cracking through a sudden change of temperature. The pail, containing a certain amount of water, is placed on the stove, the water is heated to the boiling point, the pail being then removed. The rack of bottles containing the milk preparation, with corks of non-absorbent cotton, is placed in it and the lid applied. The apparatus is placed away from a direct current of air for about forty-five minutes.

As the water in the pail cools, the milk in the bottles grows warm until both are at the same temperature. After forty-five minutes, cold water is turned into the pail to cool the bottles rapidly. They are then kept on ice until again warmed ready for use.

This is the simplest and best way to pasteurize milk and the expense is small.

Improvised apparatus may be used, but it requires much more labor and is not as satisfactory.

All milk should be sterilized or pasteurized before being used as a food for infants.

The following table shows an analysis of milks and infant foods helpful in the selection of a food to supply deficiencies indicated by a chemical analysis of the infant.

COMPARATIVE ANALYSIS OF MILKS AND INFANT FOODS (COMPILED)

(Percentage of Composition of the Dry Substance)

COMPONENTS	Mother's Milk	Cow's Milk	Borden's Malted Milk	Horlick's Malted Milk	Borden's Condensed Milk (Eagle Brand)	Nestle's Food (Milk Substitute)	Mellin's Food (Milk Modifier)	Eskay's Food (Milk Modifier)
Protein	14.00	27.00	15.10	13.83	10.10	12.40	12.10	6.82
Fat	31.00	31.00	9.20	7.90	12.10	4.15	0.25	3.58
Cane-Sugar	None	None	None	None	59.1	22.10	None	None
Other Soluble Carbohydrates (Lactose, Maltose, etc.)	52.00[1]	36.00[1]	69.77[2]	66.56[2]	16.0[1]	35.00[1]	84.00[2]	56.78[3]
Starch	None	None	None	None	None	25.70	None	30.42
Ash (Mineral Content)	2.00	5.00	3.46	3.42	2.4	1.62	3.78	1.00

[1] All lactose (milk-sugar).

[2] Mostly maltose (a hard, crystalline sugar formed by the action of malt on starch).

[3] Mostly lactose.

The following table from Holt shows at a glance the comparative average composition of human and cow's milk:

HUMAN AND COW'S MILK COMPARED

	Human Milk	Cow's Milk
Fat..........................	4%	4%
Sugar........................	7%	4.5%
Proteins.....................	1.5%	3.5%
Salts........................	0.2%	0.75%
Water........................	87.30%	87.25%
Total....................	100.00%	100.00%

Barley, rice, oatmeal, corn meal and soy-bean flour are generally used. If the grains **Gruels** of the cereals are used, they must be cooked from three to four hours.

As a rule, cereal gruels are made by cooking the flour and water for from fifteen to twenty minutes. Two ounces to the quart is about as strong as plain gruels can be made.

Dextrinized gruels may be made as high as eight ounces to the quart. Four level tablespoonfuls of the cereal flour weigh one ounce.

As the soy bean contains no starch, it does not thicken when cooking.

About 1 level tablespoonful to 3 ounces of soy-bean flour are used to the quart. One or 2 tablespoonfuls of barley, oat, or wheat gruel may be added before cooking to increase the nutritive value. One ounce of soy-bean flour, or 2 ounces of barley flour, to 1 quart of water makes a very good standard gruel. It con-

tains 2 per cent. protein, 0.6 per cent. fat, 5.1 per cent.
carbohydrates, giving a food value of ten c_lories per
ounce, just one-half the value of milk.   In certain
forms of intestinal trouble in which cow's milk is not
assimilated, this gruel is valuable used with condensed
milk.

Malted gruels are made by adding 1 teaspoonful of
good malt extract or diastase to a cereal gruel after
it has been cooled.   It should be stirred in very
thoroughly.

Vomiting	In artificial feeding "spitting" is usually
an annoying symptom that does not in-
dicate anything more serious than an overloaded
stomach. This condition is usually relieved by
lengthening the feeding intervals to four hours.

On the other hand, vomiting usually indicates something more serious in a bottle-fed baby, especially if it
is very persistent.   It is usually a sign that cow's
milk, or the preparation of it, is not agreeing with the
infant.   It also indicates a digestive disturbance that
should be treated only by the physician, who will
probably change the formula.

Occasional vomiting is sometimes due to too rich
food and too frequent feeding. Lengthening the
feeding hours and decreasing the amount of fat in
the mixture will usually eliminate the trouble.

Colic	This is the most common of all of baby's
troubles.   It is often due to too rapid feeding either from the breast or bottle, and when there is
a tendency to colic, the feeding should be slower.   The
baby should not be fed while it is suffering from colic,
even though it seems that the drinking of warm milk

relieves it temporarily. Hot water should be given
every half-hour or hour until relieved. If the baby
seems cold, hot water slightly sweetened, and a hot
bath, should be given at once. A hot-water bottle
may be placed near it as well.

In colic there is severe pain in the abdomen, which
is swollen and hard. Sudden and violent crying is
usually a symptom of colic, which often ceases very
suddenly after the emission of gas from the mouth or
bowels.

If the baby seems exhausted, the physician should
be summoned at once, but these suggestions may
be helpful until the physician arrives.

When colic is very frequent in a bottle-fed baby,
the food should be modified.

The character of the stools depends
primarily on the composition of the food. **The Stools
in Infancy**
They are varied according to the digestive
powers of the infant, and according to the amount and
rapidity of absorption of the products of digestion.
The amount of absorption depends to a considerable
extent on the rapidity with which the contents pass
through the intestinal tract.

The nature of the food, of course, influences the
character of the stools. The examination of the stools
is of the greatest aid in determining whether or not
any given food element is properly digested and assimilated, and, in many diseased conditions, in telling
what element is at fault. This, however, can only be
determined by analysis, but a little information on this
subject will be of value to the mother or nurse.

During the first few weeks or months of life, the

breast-fed infant has three or four stools daily.
These are of about the consistency of thick pea soup
and are golden yellow. The number of stools gradually diminishes to two or three in the twenty-four
hours, and the consistency becomes more salve-like.

It is not uncommon for thriving breast-fed babies
to have a large number of stools of diminished consistency and of a brownish color; in such instances,
the examination of the breast milk will show that the
proteins are high.

It is best not to pay too much attention to the
stools if the baby is gaining in weight and appears well.
It is not unusual to find many soft fine curds and
sometimes mucus in the stools of healthy breast-fed
babies.

It is not only unnecessary, but decidedly wrong to
wean a baby simply because the stools are abnormal,
if it is doing well in other ways. The breast-fed infant
will often go weeks or months without a normal stool
and yet thrive perfectly. On the other hand, if a
baby has such stools when it is taking cow's milk it is
a decided evidence of malnutrition.

Infants that are thriving on cow's milk have, as a
general rule, fewer movements in the twenty-four
hours than do breast-fed babies and these movements
are firmer in consistency.

Constipation Constipation seems to be the chief difficulty in artificial feeding, due usually to
the poor absorption of fat, or the low percentage necessary to prevent indigestion. If the constipation is
not severe, the substitution of oatmeal for barley
water in the mixture will usually relieve the trouble.

If the constipation is severe, causing occasional

attacks of colic or straining at stool, it is sometimes advisable to give a little higher percentage of fat in the mixture, but this should be done very cautiously and usually on the advice of the physician.

If, however, this does not relieve the trouble, the best plan is to substitute one of the dextrin-maltose mixtures for milk-sugar or cane-sugar. The malt itself is not especially laxative but it prevents the excessive fermentation which usually occurs when the bowels are very costive.

Two, three, or more green and loose **Diarrhea** evacuations, even though they may contain whitish particles of undigested fat, are of no great significance in the breast-fed infant, but should be regarded as danger signals in bottle-fed babies.

Even a mild attack of diarrhea is usually a symptom of fat-dyspepsia which, if taken in time, may usually be promptly checked.

A dose of castor-oil at the beginning of the attack may relieve any irritation that might have caused the trouble.

It is best to omit all food for at least twenty-four hours. Plain water should be given very freely and occasionally barley water, if the baby is hungry. After that it is best to start with a mixture low in fat. Skimmed milk or boiled milk free from all fat, diluted with cereal water, may be given at regular intervals.

Should slight diarrheal attacks continue, or should the stools be of a diarrheal character, the wisest plan is to substitute a dextrin-maltose mixture for the sugar, as malt decidedly favors fat absorption.

In almost every case of infantile diarrhea it is

advisable to consult the physician, especially if there is considerable restlessness and rise in temperature.

Diarrhea is more frequent in summer among bottle-fed babies, as the heat often promotes the growth of germs in the milk. Therefore to sterilize or pasteurize milk during the heated months is especially necessary.

A chill, due to insufficient clothing, will sometimes cause diarrhea. The abdomen, arms, and legs should be kept warm by close-fitting garments of soft wool.

Anemia   In treating anemia in infants, as in adults, the cause should be removed by correcting any errors in diet and treating any other physical deficiencies.

The cause of infantile anemia is an insufficient absorption of iron from the food.

The amount of iron in both human milk and cow's milk is small and is insufficient for the needs of the growing infant. However, Nature has deposited enough iron in the liver of the new-born infant to last until it can digest foods which contain iron in sufficient amounts. The iron in human milk is apparently more easily retained than that in the milk of animals.

The iron content of human milk is dependent on the general condition of the mother. It is higher in healthy individuals and lower in those under par.

Anemia in infants is apt to become severe and often take on a pernicious form. A prolonged intestinal disturbance often brings on anemia, and not infrequently anemia is due to a deficiency of protein in the food.

The treatment consists largely of additions or

changes in the diet, depending on the age of the infant. Purées of vegetables that contain much iron, such as spinach and carrots, and also fruit juices, are valuable and in proper proportions can be added to the diet after the age of six months. It is best that the physician decide on the advisability of this as it will depend on the general condition of the infant.

Rickets, a chronic impairment of nutrition, affects not only the bones, but all of **Rickets** the tissues of the body, particularly the nervous system. Artificial feeding is the chief cause of rickets on account of the poor absorption of fats, and often because of protein starvation.

Prepared foods, on account of their large percentage of starch and their lack of protein and butter-fat are frequently the cause of rickets.

In addition to its fuel value, milk-fat contains the elements which promote growth.

As previously stated, the infant requires a certain percentage of protein, fat, and mineral for the blood and tissue building and the growth of the bones. In artificial feeding, the preparations given are often deficient in these important elements.

Climate and poor hygienic surroundings sometimes cause rickets in breast-fed babies, probably on account of the lowered vitality of the mother and the child and consequently poor digestion and assimilation, but it is most frequently found in babies improperly fed.

Dr. Winfield S. Hall says:

Fresh milk, appropriately modified and in proper amount, together with such other food as is indicated for the age and weight, is the important point in the treatment of rickets. **Fresh air**, day and night, sunshine and outdoor life, are only next in happiness. Cod-liver oil, especially with the addition of phosphorus, is a very valuable addition to the treatment.

Scurvy   Rickets is a chronic condition, while scurvy is an acute disease.

This difficulty is considered as entirely due to improper feeding and therefore must be overcome by a change of diet. Recovery is usually very rapid when the child is properly fed.

Pains and tenderness about the joints, particularly of the legs, are the usual symptoms, causing the baby to cry when it is lifted or moved about. The gums sometimes become swollen and bleed. In almost every case it is found that infants suffering from scurvy have been on a continuous diet of prepared foods like malted milk, condensed milk, or boiled milk which Dr. Hall terms "dead food," presumably on account of a lack of the life-giving proteins and butter-fat.

When boiled milk has been used, the change should be made to pasteurized milk or raw milk if it can be secured clean and fresh. If prepared foods have been given, the amount should be greatly decreased and replaced by a cow's-milk preparation in which a small percentage of the prepared food may be included, or, better still, omitted entirely, if a cow's-milk preparation including a good substantial gruel will agree.

In scurvy, orange juice or other fruit juices should be given, from 1 to 4 ounces a day, according to the age. Orange juice is particularly valuable, 2 or 3 teaspoonfuls being given before each feeding.

A lack of fresh air often aids in producing scurvy.

After the baby has reached the age of
one year, we often feel that it is not necessary to be so careful of its diet. However,
the number of deaths due to digestive
disturbances caused by improper feeding
during the second year is significant.

After the child is a year old it should be given solid
food *very gradually* to develop its digestive functions
as well as its teeth. A soft-boiled egg or a little beef
juice may be added to the diet. Until the appearance
of the anterior molar teeth, however, the child's diet
should be confined largely to milk. A thin slice of
buttered bread or a little plain rice or rice pudding, a
soda cracker or bread crumbs in milk may be given.
The year-old child may also begin to drink cow's milk.
One or two glasses a day may be given, until the child
is at least 13 or 14 years old.

Good judgment should be used in feeding children,
as habits and tastes are being formed, and whether
they are normal or abnormal will depend on the kind
of food given and when.

Four meals a day, at regular intervals, and nothing
but water between these intervals, is considered the
best plan.

Dry toast, zwieback, and crackers may be gradually
added to the diet, also well-cooked cereals, like cream
of wheat, rice, and oatmeal. The oatmeal should be
strained the first few months it is given. Very little
sugar should be added to the cereals, as children very
quickly cultivate a desire for sweets, rejecting other
more nourishing foods, and too much sugar is apt to
disturb the digestion. It is best during the first few
months that no sugar be added to cereals.

The amount of whole milk, or milk diluted with

23

barley or oatmeal gruel, should be limited to one quart when the other foods are given.

Beef juice (from one to two ounces), mutton broth, chicken broth, and cereal broths may be given after the age of one year; not more than two ounces at first, gradually increasing in a few months' time to four ounces. This is best given at the beginning of the noon feeding. These broths have little nutritive value, but usually stimulate the appetite for other foods.

The child must build muscle, bone, and sinew, and more protein is required as soon as he begins to walk. Milk, eggs, and cereals will furnish this. The heavier protein diet is best given at eighteen months to two years, in eggs, cooked soft. An egg may be given every other day, soft boiled for about two minutes, or coddled for four minutes. At the age of two years an egg may be given every day. These soft-cooked eggs are best when mixed with broken dry toast or broken whole wheat or Graham crackers, because if dry food is served with them they will be better masticated, hence more saliva be mixed with them.

The habit of thorough mastication should be cultivated at this period.

Oatmeal, thoroughly cooked, and shredded wheat, with cream and sugar, ripe fruit, bread and butter, milk, soft-cooked eggs (poached or boiled), constitute a rational diet at this age.

Bread is better broken in milk because the chewing movements mix the saliva with the milk and smaller curds are formed as the milk enters the stomach.

Custard may after two years be added to the diet, also baked or mashed potato, plain boiled macaroni, also a little butter on the potato, toast, or bread.

Also after the age of eighteen months, a small quantity of very lean meat, like scraped or chopped beef or lamb, or finely minced chicken, may be given once a day.

Also well-cooked and mashed vegetables like peas, spinach, carrots, and asparagus tips. For the first few months these should be strained.

Some fruit should also be given each day, orange juice, apple sauce, or the pulp of stewed prunes; the latter especially is valuable when the bowels are inclined to be constipated.

Tea, coffee, and cocoa are absolutely objectionable, and before the age of two years no kind of candy should be given.

One of the most important things to teach the child, when it is taking foods other than milk, is thorough mastication, not only to assist the proper growth of the teeth, but to prevent the digestive disturbances that invariably occur from the bolting of food, and children are especially liable to do this.

Dry toast and zwieback compel mastication and strengthen the gums. These should be given in the hand, a piece at mealtime and occasionally between meals, if the child seems hungry. The child will then gradually get into the habit of chewing other solid foods when they are given.

If the child is hungry between meals, he should be fed at a regular period, midway between breakfast and luncheon and between luncheon and the evening meal. The food should be dry (toast or a dry cracker) to induce thorough and slow mastication.

Many object to "piecing" between meals, but if this piecing be done at hours as regular as his meal hour, and the food be dry and well masticated, it will readily digest and will not interfere with his meals. The growing child needs more frequent meals than the adult. His stomach is not so large, he is active in outdoor exercise, and eliminates waste freely. He also requires much heat and energy. The active child at outdoor play uses almost as much energy as the laboring man.

Many mothers are in doubt as to whether the baby's food should be salted. It is necessary to add a very little salt to the food for the baby; broths should be seasoned slightly and a pinch of salt added to potatoes and eggs. Cereals and vegetables are cooked in water to which a little salt has been added.

Experienced observers of children and their ailments and diseases have said that more babies are killed by overfeeding than by underfeeding. Especially in summer, when the child's condition reflects that of the mother, too much food will cause indigestion, irritation of the stomach, and diarrhea.

Often the child is fretful because it is too warm or is thirsty. It will often be benefited by giving it less food and more water. This fretful mind affects the child's digestion just as it affects the digestion of the mother.

If a healthy child refuses good, wholesome food because it wishes some other than what is offered it, it is not hungry and doesn't need the food.

The growing child craves sweets, but a child should not be given candy whenever it wants it during the day. Candy or sugar is quickly converted into heat and is best eaten immediately following a meal. Sugar may be spread on bread for the four o'clock lunch or a little candy may be eaten at this time. Two or three pieces of candy an inch square are sufficient.

APPENDIX

MEASURES AND WEIGHTS

A few tables of measures may be helpful here because accurate measurements are necessary to insure success in the preparation of any article of food.

All dry ingredients, such as flour, meal, powdered sugar, etc., should be sifted before measuring.

The standard measuring cup contains one-half pint and is divided into fourths and thirds.

To measure a cupful or spoonful of dry ingredients, fill the cup or spoon and then level off with the back of a case-knife.

In measures of weight the gram is the unit.

A "heaping cupful" is a level cup with two table-spoonfuls added.

A "scant cupful" is a level cup with two table-spoonfuls taken out.

A "saltspoon" is one-fourth of a level teaspoon.

To measure butter, lard, and other solid foods, pack solidly in spoon or cup and level with a knife.

TABLE OF MEASURES AND WEIGHTS[1]

4 saltspoons......................	= 1 teaspoon, tsp.
3 teaspoons.......................	= 1 tablespoon, tbsp.
4 tablespoons.....................	= ¼ cup or ½ gill.
16 tablespoons (dry ingredients)........	= 1 cup, c.

[1] *Practical Dietetics*, Alida Frances Pattee.

357

12 tablespoons (liquid)................	= 1 cup.
2 gills.............................	= 1 cup.
2 cups.............................	= 1 pint.
2 pints............................	= 1 quart.
4 quarts...........................	= 1 gallon.
2 tablespoons butter................	= 1 ounce.
1 tablespoon melted butter..........	= 1 ounce.
4 tablespoons flour.................	= 1 ounce.
2 tablespoons granulated sugar.......	= 1 ounce.
2 tablespoons liquid................	= 1 ounce.
2 tablespoons powdered lime.........	= 1 ounce.
1 cup of stale bread crumbs..........	= 2 ounces.
1 square Baker's unsweetened chocolate	= 1 ounce.
Juice of one lemon = (about) 3 table-spoons	
5 tablespoons liquid................	= 1 wineglassful.
4 cups of sifted flour...............	= 1 pound.
2 cups of butter (packed solidly)......	= 1 pound.
2 cups of finely chopped meat (packed solidly)........................	= 1 pound.
2 cups of granulated sugar...........	= 1 pound.
2⅖ cups of powdered sugar...........	= 1 pound.
2⅔ cups brown sugar................	= 1 pound.
2⅔ cups oatmeal...................	= 1 pound.
4¾ cups rolled oats.................	= 1 pound.
9 or 10 eggs.......................	= 1 pound.
1 cup of rice......................	= ½ pound.

APOTHECARIES' WEIGHTS[1]

20 grains..........................	= 1 scruple, ℈
3 scruples.........................	= 1 drachm, ℨ
8 drachms (or 480 grains)...........	= 1 ounce, ℥
12 ounces.........................	= 1 pound, lb.

APOTHECARIES' MEASURES[1]

60 minims (M).....................	= 1 fluid drachm, f℥
8 fluid drachms....................	= 1 fluid ounce, f℥
16 fluid ounces....................	= 1 pint, o or pt.
2 pints...........................	= 1 quart, qt.
4 quarts..........................	= 1 gallon, gal.

[1] *Practical Dietetics*, Alida Frances Pattee.

Appendix

APPROXIMATE MEASURES[1]

One teaspoonful.................equals about 1 fluid drachm.
One dessertspoonful..............equals about 2 fluid drachms.
One tablespoonful...............equals about 4 fluid drachms.
One wineglassful................equals about 2 ounces.
One cup (one-half pint)...........equals about 8 ounces.

METRIC MEASURES OF WEIGHT[1]

In measures of weight the gram is the unit.

1 gram.......................	1.0	gm.
1 decigram....................	0.1	gm.
1 centigram..................	0.01	gm.
1 milligram...................	0.001	gm.

[1] *Practical Dietetics*, Alida Frances Pattee.

INDEX

www.ingramcontent.com/pod-product-compliance
Lightning Source LLC
Chambersburg PA
CBHW031457270326
41930CB00006B/134